National Nursing Centers Consortium Guide

Nurse-Managed Wellness Centers

About the Editors

Tine Hansen-Turton, MGA, JD

Tine Hansen-Turton is known to be an effective change agent, systems-thinker, and policy advocate. She has over 15 years of experience in providing executive management and for the past decade she has led the National Nursing Centers Consortium (NNCC), a national movement of nurse-managed health and wellness centers serving over 2.5 million people. Dr. Hansen-Turton also serves as Vice President for Public Health Management Corporation (PHMC), a nonprofit public health institute, where she oversees several trade associations and non-profit organizations. She is an adjunct faculty member at La Salle University School of Nursing and she writes and publishes for many peer-review professional health care and legal journals.

Mary Ellen T. Miller, PhD, RN

Mary Ellen T. Miller is an Assistant Professor at De Sales University School of Nursing in Center Valley, Pennsylvania, and teaches in the undergraduate and graduate programs. Dr. Miller serves as the Co-Chair of the Wellness Center Committee of the National Nursing Centers Consortium. She is also co-director of a federal grant at La Salle University Neighborhood Nursing Center, located in Philadelphia, Pennsylvania, where she served as the Associate Director of Public Health Programs and Independence Foundation Chair for three years. Her research interests focus on adolescent and paternal risk communication.

Philip A. Greiner, DNSc, RN

Philip A. Greiner is Associate Dean for Public Health and Entrepreneurial Initiatives at Fairfield University School of Nursing, Fairfield, CT, and is the Director of the Health Promotion Center (HPC). He has served as Director for 12 years. Dr. Greiner serves as the Co-Chair of the Wellness Center Committee and on the Board of the National Nursing Centers Consortium. Over the past twelve years, he has served on the Advisory Board or Board of Directors of five community organizations in the Bridgeport, CT, area. He is currently the Chair of the Board of Directors of Southwest Community Health Center and on the Boards of the Connecticut Public Health Association and the Connecticut Association of Public Health Nurses.

National Nursing Centers Consortium Guide

Nurse-Managed Wellness Centers: Developing and Maintaining Your Center

Tine Hansen-Turton, MGA, JD
Mary Ellen T. Miller, PhD, RN
Philip A. Greiner, DNSc, RN
Editors

Managing Editor: Ann C. Deinhardt, MSW

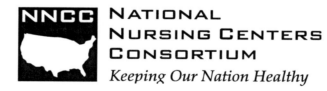

NATIONAL NURSING CENTERS CONSORTIUM
Keeping Our Nation Healthy

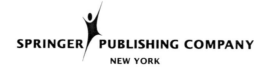

SPRINGER PUBLISHING COMPANY
NEW YORK

Springer Publishing Company, LLC
11 West 42nd Street
New York, NY 10036
www.springerpub.com

Acquisitions Editor: Allan Graubard
Cover design: David Levy
Composition: Monotype, LLC

Ebook ISBN: 978-0-8261-2133-2
09 10 11 12 / 5 4 3 2 1

Library of Congress Cataloging-in-Publication Data

Nurse-managed wellness centers : developing and maintaining your center / [edited by] Tine Hansen-Turton, Mary Ellen Miller, Phil Greiner.
   p. ; cm.
  Includes bibliographical references and index.
  ISBN 978-0-8261-2132-5
  1. Community health nursing. 2. Clinics. I. Hansen-Turton, Tine. II. Miller, Mary Ellen, PhD. III. Greiner, Phil. IV. National Nursing Centers Consortium.
  [DNLM: 1. Community Health Nursing—organization & administration—United States. 2. Community Health Centers—organization & administration—United States. 3. Fitness Centers—United States. 4. Health Promotion—United States. 5. Medically Underserved Area—United States. WY 106 N9737 2009]
RT98.N8516 2009
610.73'43—dc22
                                        2009005225

Printed in the United States of America by Hamilton Printing

Table of Contents

Section I: Introduction and Overviews

Section II: Development and Planning

Section III: Wellness Center Services

Section IV: Student Learning

Section V: Improving and Measuring Quality in Wellness Centers

Contributors

Julie Cousler Emig, MSW, LSW
Vice President, Health Promotion & Wellness
Congreso de Latinos Unidos

Diane Haleem, PhD, RN
Chair and Associate Professor
Marywood University, Department of Nursing and Public Administration

Sormeh Harounzadeh
RN Candidate
University of Pennsylvania School of Nursing

Evelyn R. Hayes, PhD, FNP-BC
Professor and Director, UD Nursing Center
University of Delaware School of Nursing

Susan M. Hinck, PhD, RN
Robert Wood Johnson Health Policy Fellow
RWJ Health Policy Fellowships Program

Penny Killian, MSN, RN, MHPNP
Assistant Clinical Professor
Drexel University, College of Nursing and Health Professions

Eunice S. King, PhD, RN
Independence Foundation
Philadelphia, PA

Maureen Leonardo, MN, CRNP, CNE, FNP-BC
Associate Professor and Manager, St. Justin Plaza
Duquesne University School of Nursing

Esther Levine-Brill, PhD, ANP-BC
Professor of Nursing
Long Island University School of Nursing, Brooklyn Campus

Rita J. Lourie, MSN, MPH, RN
Assistant Professor
Temple University, College of Health Professions

Joan F. Miller, PhD, CRNP, FNP-C
Assistant Professor and Director, Nursing Wellness Center
Bloomsburg University, McCormick Center for Human Services

Lisa Ann Plowfield, PhD, RN
Dean College of Nursing
Florida State University, College of Nursing

Lenore (Leni) K. Resick, PhD, CRNP, FNP-BC, NP-C
Associate Professor and Director, DUSON Nurse-Managed Wellness Center
Duquesne University School of Nursing

Nancy L. Rothman, EdD, RN
Independence Foundation Chair of Urban Community Health Nursing
Temple University, College of Health Professions

M. Elaine Tagliareni, EdD, RN
Professor/Independence Foundation Chair
Community College of Philadelphia, Department of Nursing

Donna L. Torrisi, MSN, CRNP
Network Executive Director
Family Practice & Counseling Network

Foreword

Imagine a world where health care is available to everyone. A world where the focus on wellness is the point of entry to the health care system, where quality, safety, and clinical decision-making take place in partnership with individuals and communities, where social workers, psychologists, physicians, medical assistants, nutritionists, and outreach workers collaborate with advanced practice nurses to ensure high-quality programs, and you have imagined a nurse-managed wellness center. A health care home for people where the essence of care is trust, relationships, and partnering with communities to address their unique needs. This is a world where people of all ages thrive, grow, and maintain their optimum level of wellness. This is a world of health and wellness care administered and delivered by advanced nurse practitioners, faculty, and students. Wellness centers are the heart and soul of this world.

Since 1993, the Independence Foundation has embraced the world of community and wellness centers. We are proud of the work of this group. It is a shining example in the field of health care delivery. It is the safety net for so many without access to care.

In the following pages, you will read about what a nurse-managed wellness center is and how to plan for, market, fund, and measure its quality. This book is a toolkit and is meant to be used as a guide by the practitioner. It shares lessons learned and wisdom gained through personal experience, as well as standards to measure quality. It is an implementation tool—not a philosophical argument. It is meaningful, candid, honest, and visionary. This guide will get you started and keep you moving forward.

I commend the authors for their work and offer this book to you as an excellent tool for any advanced practice nurse, faculty member, or student who wants to practice in the community. This book embodies nursing's lessons at their finest.

Susan Sherman
President
Independence Foundation

Preface

With over 45 million uninsured in America, the need for accessible, affordable, quality health care has never been greater. Lack of access and insurance is no longer just the burden of the poor. People without a regular source of health care pose a costly long-term burden on the nation, so it is in both state and federal governments' interests to promote increased access to health care. Health disparities have widened, as more and more people report having little or no access to preventive services, also known as wellness services. For the past 40 years, Nurse-Managed Wellness Centers, led primarily by advanced practice nurses, have sprung up all over the country. With a prevention focus, these centers provide important health promotion and disease prevention services to all populations.

This Wellness Center book provides a step-by-step guide to starting and sustaining non-profit, academic-based, or independent Wellness Centers. The contributors share their firsthand knowledge with readers, including information on developing a Wellness Center, pulling together an advisory or governing board, writing business and strategic plans, getting funding, conducting research, and providing educational opportunities for students. The Appendices are rich with resources, including profiles of a number of wellness centers, examplars of wellness centers and wellness programs, a policy and procedure manual table of contents, job descriptions, a sample local agency contract, and tools for student programs and outcome documentation.

While not necessary, *Community and Nurse-Managed Health Centers: Getting Them Started and Keeping Them Going*, published by the NNCC and Springer Publishing Company in 2005, is a perfect companion to this Wellness Center book. For instance, it contains sample bylaws and a number of example policies and procedures, including a HIPAA procedure.

A great deal goes into writing a book such as this, especially when it is done with so many different people. Each contributor to this book presents a unique focus and puts forward critical lessons learned in developing, managing, and leading Wellness Centers. Best of all, the book is about nurses and health care leaders who are passionate about what they do and how Wellness Centers and services can play a critical role in enhancing access to care, as well as providing quality care for the people who are exposed to them.

Specifically, the book is structured into five sections with appendices. Section I provides an overview by Tine Hansen-Turton. In Chapters 2 and 3, Eunice King, Maureen Leonardo, and Lenore (Leni) Resick provide insight into the historical and current perspectives of what a wellness center is and how to incorporate the Boyer Model into professional practice. In Section II, Phil Greiner discusses some of the steps necessary to begin a wellness center

(Chapter 4), as do Maureen Leonardo, Leni Resick, and others (Chapter 5). Esther Brill, Rita Lourie, and Mary Ellen Miller suggest methods to develop and maintain community partnerships (Chapter 6). Phil Greiner returns in Chapter 7 with successful strategies for sustainability in an era of funding challenges. Donna Torrisi, Tine Hansen-Turton, and Ann Deinhardt reconfigure some pieces from NNCC's Primary Care book to address organizational development for larger centers in Chapter 8.

Section III features services that traditional wellness centers provide as surveyed, in Chapter 9, by Ann Deinhardt and Sormeh Harounzadeh, with input on Best Practices from Tine Hansen-Turton, Nancy Rothman, and others. Specific services provided to older people are highlighted by Diane Haleem in Chapter 10, and services designed to be successful with Latinos are discussed by Julie Cousler Emig in Chapter 11.The specialty of mental health services in wellness centers is addressed by Penny Killian and Roberta Waite (Chapter 12). Donna Torrisi clarifies how behavioral health services can be integrated in a wellness center (Chapter 12).

Numerous people made contributions regarding student involvement through community service and learning activities, which Section IV highlights. In Chapter 13, Diane Haleem, Evelyn Hayes, Joan Miller, Mary Ellen Miller, and Lisa Plowfield explicate Community Service and Learning (CSL) activities. Approaches for engaging youth in health careers to build nursing's future capacity are outlined by Evelyn Hayes and Lisa Plowfield in Chapter 14.

Section V discusses the necessities of improving and measuring quality. Susan Hinck in Chapter 15 informs readers of the importance of measuring quality in a wellness center model. Several strategies to document outcomes are provided by Evelyn, Maureen, Lisa, and Leni in Chapter 16. In the final chapter, Eunice King and Elaine Tagliareni discuss systems for data collection.

Acknowledgments

Acknowledgments From NNCC

The NNCC Board of Directors and I are pleased to present this Wellness Center book and toolkit, which can be used by many audiences including faculty, students, health care professionals, and various organizations interested in providing the most basic health services to people in need. The book is modeled after the NNCC's *American Journal of Nursing* award-winning guide, *Community and Nurse-Managed Health Centers: Getting Them Started and Keeping Them Going*, published by Springer Publishing Company in 2005.

This book is primarily the work of an energetic NNCC Wellness Center Committee, lead ably by Dr. Mary Ellen Miller and Dr. Phil Greiner. Over the past four years, this group has worked to provide technical assistance to many academics and others on how to provide wellness services successfully. This Wellness book is a compilation of information that over 20 Wellness Center and other health care leaders have put together to pass along their leadership experiences in managing and running successful Wellness Centers. In addition to the Wellness Center Committee, special thanks go to the NNCC Mental Health Task Force and a number of others, who also contributed, and to Ann Deinhardt, who assisted with the previous book and managed the task of bringing this one together. Sormeh Harounzadeh, a student who worked at NNCC for the summer of 2008, and Brian Valdez also provided valuable assistance in the development of this book. We are especially grateful to Susan Sherman, President and CEO, and Judge Phyllis Beck, Board Chair of the Independence Foundation, for continuing to be our fortress and continuing to invest energy and resources into nurse-managed health and wellness centers and the National Nursing Centers Consortium. The steadfast commitment to ensuring that all people have access to wellness services is truly amazing.

Finally, we salute all staff and students who work in the NNCC and the Wellness Centers and patients for putting their faith in a different kind of community model of care.

Tine Hansen-Turton, MGA, JD
CEO, National Nursing Centers Consortium

Acknowledgments From Wellness Committee Co-Chairs

In 2004, we discussed with Tine Hansen-Turton, the CEO of NNCC, the feasibility of initiating a committee that would serve exclusively the needs of nurse-managed wellness centers. At the time, we both were directors of academic wellness centers, so Tine and the Board were very support- ive of this initiative and suggested that we partner to co-chair a Well- ness Committee. Over the next two years, this Committee evolved into a vibrant group of professionals from throughout the United States. Mem- bership is comprised of wellness center directors, public health nurses, and adjunct faculty who engage in practice in wellness centers. Monthly meetings are conducted via conference calls and meeting minutes are sent to all members by Brian Valdez, NNCC Health Policy Manager, who so ably staffs the committee.

Although the Wellness Committee members wear many hats in their respective centers, one commonality that surfaced early was that all mem- bers had not only expertise, but "lessons learned along the way" to share with colleagues from other wellness centers. To accomplish this, Wellness Committee members partnered to submit abstracts for presentations at the NNCC Annual Best Practice Conference in 2006, and again in 2007. Their goal was to share national best practices in wellness centers, as well as to assist other professionals from academia and public health to either establish or sustain wellness centers. Feedback from participants at both conferences was overwhelmingly positive. A common theme that emerged from evaluation surveys was that there was a need for even more "practical" information that could be used in participants' home organizations, includ- ing job descriptions and strategies to involve students.

The inspiration for this book evolved from an informal de-briefing session immediately following the 2007 NNCC Conference, where Well- ness Committee members brainstormed ways to meet the varied needs expressed by the conference participants. The group discussed the utility of the NNCC book, *Community and Nurse-Managed Health Centers: Getting Them Started and Keeping Them Going*, by Donna Torrisi and Tine Hansen-Turton, which focuses on primary care nurse-managed centers. All believed that a publication based upon this model, but addressing the unique needs of wellness centers, would be a valuable tool for those who are actively engaged in or contemplating starting up a wellness center. By aiding in the establishment or sustaining of wellness centers, the communities served would be the beneficiaries in the long term. As Wellness Commit- tee co-chairs, we approached Tine shortly after the conference about the feasibility of developing a "Wellness Center" book. She wholeheartedly supported this endeavor and began to explore a publishing opportunity with Springer Publishing Company. Tine continues to be a steadfast ally of wellness centers internationally. We are extremely grateful to her for keeping us on track with timelines, as well as for her editorial feedback.

The Wellness Committee members and other professionals who sacrificed time from their families and work commitments to contribute to this book are worthy of note. The articles are collaborative works contributed by Wellness Committee members and others who are content specialists in their respective topical areas. This book is a "snapshot" of their contributions to wellness centers. It is not humanly possible to place their critical thinking skills, personal expertise, business savvy, student mentorship aptitude, and ability to build and maintain relationships into written format. It is our intention that this book will serve to aid those who are passionate about community health and wellness and assist them to improve the quality of life for those they serve in wellness centers around the country.

Mary Ellen Miller, PhD, RN
Phil Greiner, DNSc, RN

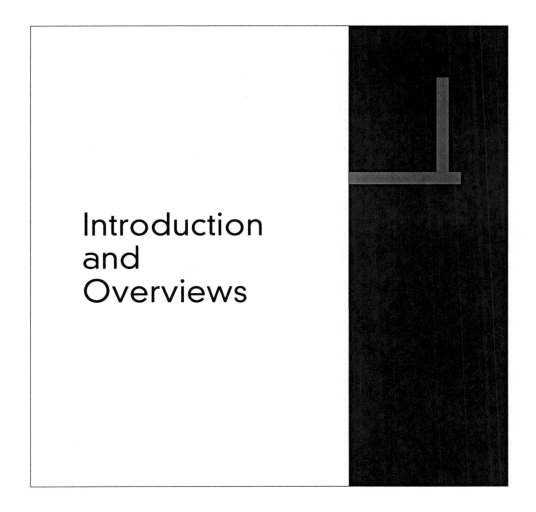

Introduction and Overviews

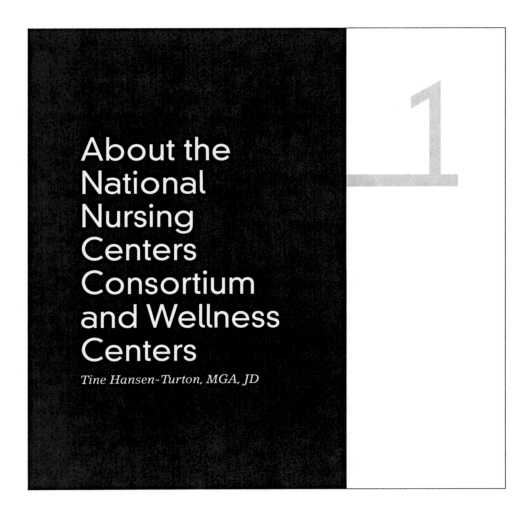

About the National Nursing Centers Consortium and Wellness Centers

Tine Hansen-Turton, MGA, JD

The National Nursing Centers Consortium

We do not often hear about the places in America where health care is working. Nurse-managed health and wellness centers work because they are focused at the community level where national and state health policies and social reality meet. The National Nursing Centers Consortium (NNCC) is a national and increasingly international incubator for creative, innovative, and nontraditional approaches to health care. The NNCC was founded to provide a forum for community-based nurse-managed health and wellness centers to share best practices and address common challenges.

The NNCC, now an affiliate of the Public Health Management Corporation, a public health institute, was established in 1996. A non-profit association of nurse-managed community-based health and wellness centers in the U.S., the NNCC has the mission to strengthen the capacity, growth, and development of nurse-managed health and wellness centers to provide access to quality care for vulnerable populations and to eliminate health disparities. The goals are to provide national leadership in identifying, tracking, and advising health care policy development; to position nurse-managed health centers as a recognized, cost-effective mainstream health care model; and to foster partnerships with people and groups who share common goals.

The NNCC represents nurse-managed health and wellness centers serving vulnerable populations across the country. These centers seek to be recognized, and thus to be more effective, as an integral part of the nation's health care delivery system. NNCC's membership is comprised of over 200 centers, which together provide health promotion and disease prevention services, as well as primary health care, to over 2.5 million people. To support its membership, the NNCC has an ambitious policy and advocacy agenda. The agenda is mission driven and geared towards the sustainability of the nurse-managed health and wellness center model.

To further its mission, the NNCC develops best-practice health promotion and disease prevention programs and professional education services to address health disparities in underserved and vulnerable communities. These signature programs and education services to help people lead healthier and safer lives address such public health concerns as asthma, lead poisoning, obesity, cardiovascular disease, pre- and neonatal health, and tobacco cessation, and are administered by NNCC in partnership with its member nurse-managed centers. These programs help avert future health problems and keep health care costs from rising further and include Asthma Safe Kids, an in-home asthma management and trigger-reduction program; Lead Safe Babies, an in-home primary prevention program to prevent lead poisoning in children; the Beck Fellowship, which trains CRNPs in use of cognitive therapy; Healthy Homes, an indoor environmental health hazard assessment program; Tobacco Cessation, which offers adults counseling to end tobacco use; and Students Run Philly Style, a long-distance running and mentoring program for youth.

NNCC is proud of its decade-strong history in developing best practice programs that meet the needs of the most underserved communities, and managing disease management, health education, and primary prevention programs in partnership with its member nurse-managed health and wellness centers.

About Nurse-Managed Health and Wellness Centers

Statistics show that there are currently over 44 million Americans without health insurance, and the number is expected to grow to 55 million by the year 2010. Nurse-managed health and wellness centers directly address this problem in that approximately 50% or 500,000 of the clients receiving treatment at the centers are uninsured.

There are approximately 250 nurse-managed health and wellness centers across the nation. These centers help to reduce health disparities by providing access to a combination of health promotion and disease prevention services and high quality comprehensive primary health care to people who otherwise have minimal access to care. Health problems or potential health problems are not viewed in isolation, but within the context of societal, environmental, and cultural influences that have impacted the client's past and present health and that have the potential to impact future health. Patients are connected with resources that address and correct the forces that have negatively impacted their health. Of the 250 centers nationally, over 150 are wellness centers that focus on primary, secondary, and tertiary preventive health care. Approximately

90 of the centers also provide comprehensive primary health care services and serve as primary care providers in their communities. The majority (60%) of nurse-managed health and wellness centers are affiliated with university-based schools of nursing. The remaining centers (40%) are independent non-profits or hospital outpatient clinics.

Nursing Education and Shortage

Nurse-managed health and wellness centers present a positive image of the future of nursing and contribute to solving the national nursing shortage. Centers provide practice opportunities for faculty, training sites for students, and experiences that often lead students to choose to serve in underserved communities. In academic centers, nurse faculty members provide positive role models for the nation's future nurses along with exposure to community-based education, practice, and research. Nursing students at all levels are able to practice in vulnerable community-based settings and become part of a pool of providers from which the federal government can draw to alleviate a growing dearth of qualified providers in underserved communities across the nation.

Services Provided

In a recent study of member organizations, NNCC found that Preventive Health services constitute the largest category of services provided, followed by Reproductive Health and Behavioral Health services. Analysis revealed behavioral health problems to be the most frequent diagnosis in the centers, followed by hypertension, diabetes, asthma, and obesity. Asthma-related diagnoses represented 32% of all pulmonary diagnoses; hypertension represented 77% of all cardiovascular diagnoses; and diabetes 69% and obesity 25% of all metabolic diagnoses. These findings confirm that nurse-managed health and wellness centers directly address health disparities. Preventive health services, such as immunizations, screenings, and health education, are considered among the most critical factors in eliminating health disparities, and these are the focal point in member centers' care delivery. Further, the nurse-managed health centers integrate Behavioral Health with Primary Care services, which is another critical factor in eliminating health disparities.

Members also provide enabling services to complement preventive and primary care. These services facilitate clients' access to the health care system and assist in the maintenance of their health. Services include the provision of transportation to and from the health and specialty appointments, and outreach services that assist clients in applying for medical assistance and cash or housing assistance. The other most common enabling services are: Outreach, Home Visiting, Health Education, Parenting Education, Environmental Health Risk Reduction, Case Management, and Interpretation/Translation Services.

The NNCC survey of members found that most staff are certified registered nurse-practitioners (20%) and advanced practice nurses (23%). Other staff are RNs (9%); therapists and social workers (6.5%); community outreach workers (4%); and health educators, students, and others (25%). Providers within nurse-managed health and wellness centers view their patients as partners in care and strive to provide patients with knowledge and skills to empower them to assume responsibility for their own health, to make informed decisions about their health, and to become their own advocates.

Populations Served

Nurse-managed health and wellness centers are safety-net providers usually located in or near health professions shortage areas and medically under-served areas, including urban, rural, and suburban communities. They are found in public and Section 8 housing developments, schools, churches, community and recreation centers, and homeless and domestic violence shelters, and provide care to low income, minority, homeless and migrant families, and uninsured populations.

A 2006 survey of NNCC members found that over half of the people served are female and come from minority populations (41% African American, 12% Latino, and 11% other non-Caucasian), which are more likely to suffer health disparities. The centers serve all age groups, but many have a large focus on children and youth (36%), suggesting the centers are getting services to underserved populations at an early age and critical to providing preventive health. Under 15% of clients in member centers had gone beyond high school in their education. Of the 69,468 clients for whom employment status was reported, 54% were unemployed. However, patients who were employed were less likely to have insurance than those who were unemployed. The study suggested that many patients are unemployed women and children on Medicaid or people who are employed but do not have access to health insurance.

Outcomes

Data from Medicaid managed care organizations and recent studies demonstrate that patients receiving care at nurse-managed health centers experience significantly fewer emergency room visits, hospital inpatient days, and specialist visits, and are at significantly lower risk of giving birth to low-birth weight infants compared to patients in conventional health care. In a recent study, nurse-managed health center patients were surveyed using the Medical Outcomes Trust Patient Satisfaction tool. Analysis of questions pertaining to patient access to health care and manner of health care delivered to patients by their primary care providers showed mean aggregate scores ranging from 4.03 to 4.19 on a 5-point scale. Findings suggested that patients were satisfied with the accessibility and delivery of care at nurse-managed centers. This finding coincides with existing literature, which has shown that patients consistently rate their satisfaction with care from CRNPs as high.

In summary, nurse-managed wellness and health centers are in a unique position to be part of the solutions to the many challenges the U.S. health care system is facing.

Resources

Torrisi, D. L., & Hansen-Turton, T. (2005). *Community and Nurse-Managed Health Centers: Getting Them Started and Keeping Them Going.* New York: Springer Publishing Company.

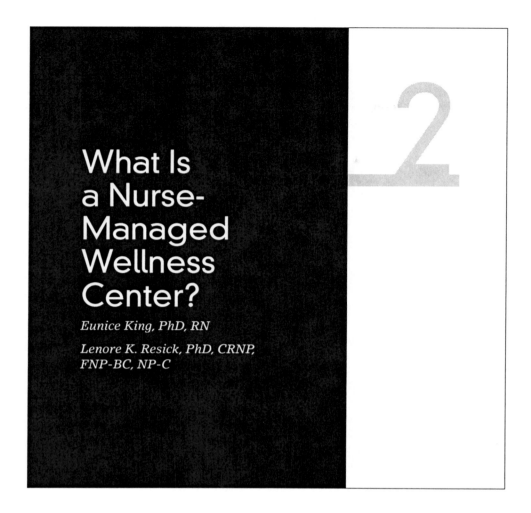

What Is a Nurse-Managed Wellness Center?

Eunice King, PhD, RN

Lenore K. Resick, PhD, CRNP, FNP-BC, NP-C

What Is a Nurse-Managed Wellness Center?

Nurse-managed wellness centers, like other models of nurse-managed centers, are community-based and are managed and staffed by registered nurses and advanced practice nurses, such as nurse-practitioners, who have advanced clinical education in a health care specialty (Torrisi & Hansen-Turton, 2005). The concept of "nurse-managed wellness" involves the management of wellness of a client by an advanced practice nurse (Resick, Taylor, & Leonardo, 1999). A characteristic unique to nurse-managed wellness centers is the primary focus on the management of wellness of an individual. Wellness center services include disease prevention, health promotion, and wellness programs. Unlike traditional primary care nursing center models, which provide a continuum of health services including both wellness and primary care services, nurse-managed wellness centers provide care that is exclusively focused on the wellness end of the continuum of health services.

In many ways, wellness centers are more like than they are unlike nursing centers that provide traditional primary care. Like traditional primary care model nursing centers, wellness centers often begin because of an invitation from the community and continue to work in partnership with the communities they serve, and they are embedded in the core of community life (Hansen-Turton & Kinsey, 2001). Nurse-managed wellness centers include the characteristics of nursing centers described by Aydelotte and others (1987) as:

> Organizations that give clients and communities direct access to professional nursing services. Professional nurses in these centers diagnose and treat human responses to actual and potential health problems, and promote health and optimal functioning among target populations and communities. The services provided in these centers are holistic, client-centered, and affordable. Overall accountability and responsibility remain with the nurse executive/director. Nurse-managed health centers are not limited to any particular organizational configuration. Nurse-managed centers can be freestanding businesses or may be affiliated with universities or other service institutions like home health agencies and hospitals. The primary characteristic of the organization is responsiveness to the health needs of populations. The nurse is responsible for all patient care and operations. (Aydelotte et al., 1987)

The wellness center model stresses health education and facilitates self-care of the individual in regard to health care strategies and decision making. Services offered by a wellness center vary and are determined by the needs of the community. Most often, these services build on the goals of *Healthy People 2000* (U.S. Department of Health and Human Services, 1991), which are to increase years of healthy living, reduce health disparities, and increase access to preventive services for all Americans. Services now focus on many of the areas identified in *Healthy People 2010* (U.S. Department of Health and Human Services, retrieved July 12, 2008). These include programs aimed at weight control, smoking cessation, physical activity and fitness, occupational safety and health, health communication, stress management, and ways to stay healthy and prevent illness such as diabetes, cancer, and HIV. An essential component to success is understanding the meaning of health and "wellness" from the perspective of the client using the services of the wellness center. This understanding is essential to the nurse-client relationship and plan of care.

Wellness centers serve urban and rural populations and are located in communities as freestanding centers or as part of other organizations such as schools, universities, and workplaces. Wellness center staff often work in conjunction with clients' traditional primary care providers to perform screening services that determine the appropriate use of health care providers so services are used appropriately and not duplicated. Although some screening services provided by nurse-managed wellness centers are reimbursable, the lack of third party reimbursement has been a challenge to maintain sustainability for many nurse-managed wellness centers not supported by ongoing grants, foundations, or a larger agency such as a school, university or workplace.

Historical Perspective

Nurses have a tradition of providing health promotion and wellness services to the general public that dates back at least to the late 19th century. In 1893, Lillian Wald established the Henry Street Nurses Settlement for the Poor and Infirm to administer to the health care needs of the poor in New York City, and around the same time, Margaret Sanger established the nation's first birth control clinic. Somewhat later, the Sheppard-Towner Act, passed during the 1920s, allocated money to states to improve the health of mothers and babies, giving public health nurses a critical role in promoting prenatal, postpartum, and infancy care. During the 1920s, Mary Breckinridge, a nurse with the Frontier Nursing Service, founded one of the earliest nursing centers — in Hayden, Kentucky — that expanded the scope of services to include midwifery and routine immunizations and check-ups for infants and preschoolers, as well as sick care and social services. By the end of 1930, there were six centers in that area, each serving a five-mile radius and financed by a $1 annual prospective payment, in either cash or goods, from every household (Glass, 1989).

During the next decade, the Social Security Act of 1935 was passed appropriating: a) money for nurses to work with state and local health departments to monitor and protect the health of the community, and, for the first time, b) funding for the training of nurses, specifically public health nurses, to fulfill this new role. Thus, many of the original nursing centers were replaced by public health nursing departments or public health divisions within municipal or county health departments. Although they continued to provide some care to the sick in the community, the focus of their work shifted to preventive services, such as administering immunizations, providing well-child checkups, conducting screening programs for communicable diseases, and tracking contacts of patients with communicable diseases, such as tuberculosis or venereal diseases. For the next several decades, wellness services were provided largely through local public health departments, but varied in nature and scope and were limited by the resources available to them.

The Division of Nursing, an organizational unit within the Bureau of Health Professions, one of the four divisions within the Health Resources and Services Administration (HRSA) of the U.S. Department of Health and Human Services, has played a very important role in the development of the nurse-managed health center model of health care delivery. Established initially as a division within the United States Public Health Services, it emerged from the United States Cadet Nurse Corps created under the Bolton Act of 1943 to relieve the severe shortage of nurses during World War II. Historically, the Division of Nursing has been the federal agency responsible for providing a national perspective on the nursing workforce, nursing practice, and nursing education. Its contributions to the nurse-managed health center movement have included: a) support for the creation of the nurse-practitioner and other advanced practice nurse roles, and b) advocacy for federal funding to develop models of care for the underserved, one of which is the nurse-managed health center. Over the next half century, a series of legislative acts were passed that provided funding to schools of nursing for the overall purposes of: a) increasing the number of nurses with baccalaureate and graduate degrees to assume positions in education and nursing, b) improving schools of nursing facilities and educational programs, c) encouraging advanced practice nursing roles, and d) increasing access to nursing resources in underserved areas (HRSA, BHP, Division of Nursing, 1997).

Another trend contributing to the development of today's nurse-managed centers, whether they offer exclusively wellness services or a combination of primary care and wellness, was that begun in the late 1970s of schools of nursing promoting clinical practice by faculty. Up until that time, many faculty members did not continue to practice once they accepted a teaching position. However, with the emergence of advanced nurse practice roles, it became critical that faculty exhibit expert clinical competence. Some schools established clinics run by nurse-practitioner or other advanced practice nursing faculty, simultaneously providing a site for faculty practice and a clinical practice site for nursing students. Between 1977 and 1979, the Division of Nursing funded clinics in a variety of settings, such as psychiatric day care centers, Head Start programs, prisons, and residential complexes for the elderly.

Through Section 3 of the Nurse Education Amendments of 1985, the Division of Nursing's Special Projects Program was reauthorized, and funds were made available for projects to improve access to nursing services in non-institutional settings. These funds have supported nurse-managed health centers established by academic schools or departments of nursing. By 1992, the Program was supporting 17 nursing centers (Starbecker, 2000). Subsequent legislation in the 1990s (i.e., the Nurse Education and Practice Improvement Amendments Act of 1992 and the Health Professions Education Partnerships Act of 1998, Public Law 105-392) emphasized the need for these centers to improve access to primary health care in medically underserved communities and to care for underserved populations (Clear, Starbecker, & Kelly, 1999; USPHS, Division of Nursing, 2000). Thus, many of the nurse-managed centers established by schools of nursing included primary care among their wellness services, but faced many challenges in achieving financial sustainability (King, 2008), and some were forced to close. Historically, there has been no reimbursement through third party payers for health promotion programs, so support for wellness programs has had to be obtained through grants from private foundations and contracts with public agencies or organizations.

One private foundation that has been an avid supporter of nurse-managed health centers is the Independence Foundation, a private, regional foundation located in Philadelphia, Pennsylvania. In 1993, its Board of Directors designated nurse-managed health care as one of its four funding priorities and, over the course of the next 12 years, awarded a total of $27,819,042 in grants that supported nurse-managed health centers. Included within that total was funding for nurse-managed health centers that offered exclusively wellness services in addition to those offering primary care as well. During that time period, 12 nurse-managed wellness centers were funded. By the end of 1999, only 3 of those 12 continued to receive funding. Of the nine centers no longer receiving Independence Foundation funding, three had either expanded their scope of services to include primary care or became part of a nursing center that did, three were not funded due to Foundation concerns about their lack of success in seeking and procuring other funding sources, and three had either closed the center or program and/or changed the mission. Since the health promotion/wellness services offered by these centers were not reimbursed by third-party payers, it became clear to the Foundation that they could survive only by cultivating multiple funding streams that might include a combination of foundations, local sources (e.g., carve out grants and contracts from local health departments), and/or HRSA's Division of Nursing, or by offering primary care and becoming eligible for third-party reimbursement. Thus, the Foundation further refined its priorities in the nurse-managed initiative to focus on those centers that included primary care (King, 2005).

In spite of this shift in priorities, the Foundation did fund two projects that directly supported the work of all nurse-managed centers, including those exclusively offering wellness services. First, the Foundation funded the Regional Nursing Centers Consortium, established in 1996 by 13 Philadelphia area nurse-managed health centers with the express mission of strengthening the capacity, growth, and development of nurse-managed health centers to enable them to provide quality health care services to vulnerable populations and to eliminate health disparities in underserved communities. By the end of 2001, membership in the RNCC had grown to 36 centers located in ten states, and the RNCC changed its name to the National Nursing Centers Consortium, consistent with the geographical dispersion of its membership and its work on behalf of nurse-managed centers throughout the United States. As of the end of 2007, over 200 centers in 40 states were members of the NNCC. Second, in recognition of the need for data to describe the scope of services provided and clients served by nurse-managed wellness centers, the Foundation awarded a series of grants to the Community College of Philadelphia to develop a data collection tool that could be used by nursing centers to document the scope of services provided and numbers of clients served. These data could be used by individual centers for report and grant proposals and could be aggregated for use by the NNCC in its efforts to procure funding for wellness programs that could be implemented by multiple centers (Tagliareni & King, 2006). (Note: For further discussion of data collection issues and description of this tool, please see Chapters 15, 16, and 17.)

Summary

Although nurse-managed wellness centers share many characteristics with nursing centers that provide traditional primary care, they are unique in their exclusive focus on the management of the wellness of their clients. Wellness center services encompass disease prevention, health promotion, and wellness programs, but the exact nature of those programs varies depending upon the needs of the community served. Funding for nurse-managed wellness centers continues to be challenging because, historically, there has been no reimbursement for health promotion programs through third-party payers. Support for wellness programs has primarily been obtained through grants and contracts with private foundations and public agencies or organizations. An immediate challenge for nurse-managed wellness centers is to demonstrate to policymakers the value of such centers and, as a result, to be included among the strategies for reforming the current health care system.

Application of the Boyer Model of Scholarship in Nurse-Managed Wellness Centers

Lenore K. Resick, PhD, CRNP, FNP-BC, NP-C
Maureen E. Leonardo, MN, CRNP, CNE, FNP-BC

Introduction

Many nurse-managed wellness centers are housed in or affiliated with academic institutions. The individuals who are managing or working in these wellness centers are often faculty who teach in the classroom and the clinical arena and maintain a clinical practice through the centers. These faculty need to show evidence of scholarly work for the purpose of promotion and tenure. So the questions arise: Does their work within the wellness center reflect scholarship? How can it be used for promotion and tenure? The purpose of this chapter is to describe the Boyer Model of Scholarship, which interprets scholarship in a broader context, and illustrate the application of its components at one nurse-managed wellness center with evidence of scholarly work.

The Boyer Model of Scholarship

In a report written in 1990 titled *Scholarship Reconsidered: Priorities of the Professoriate,* Boyer wrote that if institutions of higher learning are to continue to advance, there needs to be an expanded vision of the definition and understanding of scholarship. He wrote that there is a mismatch in the practice of universities who hire professors to teach, but then evaluate them based on the production and dissemination of research. Within this paradigm, teaching is not valued or considered as the priority over research and dissemination of research. Although hired to teach, survival of the professors in academia is directly related to their engagement in research, publication, and presentation, not the amount or quality of the teaching they are hired to do. Most universities require faculty to be engaged in research, teaching, and service. Boyer made the argument that, if institutions of higher learning are to continue to advance, a new understanding and definition of what constitutes scholarship is needed and that, although valued, research alone is insufficient to prepare the next generation for the future.

To address the new definition of what constitutes scholarship, Boyer described four types: discovery, integration, application, and teaching. Each type of scholarship is separate but they overlap, and all should be rewarded.

Description and Application of the Four Types of Scholarship

The scholarship of discovery, or research, has traditionally been the gold standard of academic achievement and brings financial incentives to the university and school. Discovery of new knowledge through traditional research methods involves the creative process and adds to the intellectual environment of the university. Traditionally, assessment of discovery involves dissemination of findings by peer-reviewed presentations and publications (Nibert, n.d.).

Boyer described the scholarship of integration as giving meaning to isolated facts. It is closely related to the scholarship of discovery. This type of scholarship involves collaboration and synthesis. It involves interpreting and seeing problems from many perspectives, including across disciplines, and coordinating one's own research interest with others into a large woven pattern of intellectual design. The scholarship of integration is very natural for a nursing center since nursing centers are often places where many disciplines converge. That is, nursing centers are a natural place for multidisciplinary approaches toward the common goal of wellness. There may be challenges in implementing integration, such as conflicting times of clinical schedules/hours, research agendas of competing departments or universities, competition for limited funding sources, and turf issues.

The scholarship of application involves "service" from the perspective of engagement. It involves theory to practice to solve common problems and challenges resulting in scholarly engagement. Although most universities consider service as part of the "teaching, research, service" triad, and a requirement of an academic appointment, the value of service depends to a large extent on the mission of the institution. It should, however, be considered an act of scholarship on par with discovery, integration, and teaching. In order for this to occur, it is important to "distinguish applied scholarship (professional service or outreach) from campus and community citizenship" (Glassick, Huber, & Maeroff, 1997, p. 12). Service activities that are scholarly must be tied directly to one's special field and flow directly from it.

Lastly, the scholarship of teaching involves teaching that models the highest values of the profession. Students are taught to comprehend and synthesize theory. Ideally, this type of scholarship includes reflection and is open to evaluation and feedback that ideally contribute to improvement of teaching for the profession. In addition, students learn and develop a passion for scholarship. Learning from student feedback enriches teaching.

Application of the Boyer Model

As the gold standard of academic achievement, the scholarship of discovery may be applied using traditional methods of research in nursing centers. There still remains a paucity of research on wellness, especially in vulnerable or underserved populations such as those served by the wellness centers.

Nursing centers based on a wellness model can provide a rich environment for experimenting with various modes of care delivery, especially the interventions of the advanced practice nurse that are purely nursing interventions. Although several studies address the medical model and interventions by advanced practice nurses, few studies have researched the interventions of advanced practice nurses that are purely nursing (Fiandt, Laux, Sarver, & Sayer, 2002).

The scholarship of integration is natural for a nursing center since nursing centers are often the place where many disciplines converge; that is, nursing centers are a natural place for multidisciplinary approaches to the common goal of wellness. Some of the scholarly activities that support integration include the preparation of an extensive and comprehensive review of literature; authoring a multidisciplinary text book; collaboration in course design, especially cross-discipline, and course implementation; and the development of interdisciplinary, evidence-based clinical activity (Nilbert, n.d.; Glassick, et al., 1997).

With regard to nursing wellness centers, the scholarship of application involves leaving the classroom and going with the students into the field where real life situations are encountered and faculty and students seek to discover how academia can help solve problems of health care and social issues in general. In order to be applied, the knowledge has to first have been discovered. This type of research involves working with the unknown, being comfortable with "not knowing", and seeking ways that knowledge can be applied to practice. Scholarly activities that address the scholarship of application include assuming a leadership role in professional organizations, taking on the role of a professional model for students, and serving as an external consultant for both industry and governmental agencies (Nibert, n.d.).

Teaching is central to scholarship and not only requires knowledge and articulation of the subject but also creativity to invent methods to communicate this knowledge. Human experience is extremely valuable to the learning process and is the focus of the nursing center experience. Examples of the scholarship of teaching include classroom research and the advancement of learning theory; the creation, testing, or evaluation of instructional materials; the mentoring of students; and the design and implementation of a program evaluation plan (Nibert, n.d.).

Implementation in a Nurse-Managed Wellness Center

Implementation of the Boyer Model means new expectations of faculty and rethinking the way faculty are recognized and how their performance is evaluated. Not all academic institutions have mission statements and faculty handbook policies that support the interpretation of the four aspects of the Boyer Model as scholarship. Knowledge of the mission statement of the academic institution and the faculty handbook concerning tenure and promotion and the criteria considered as scholarship are important considerations for faculty who are planning to devote time to planning, implementing, and evaluating a nurse-managed wellness center. Clinical faculty may find it necessary to take a proactive stance and provide academic administration, faculty senate, and the tenure and promotion review board of the academic institution with a rationale for consideration of using the Boyer Model as an evaluation of teaching and scholarship.

The writers of this chapter successfully progressed through the promotion and tenure process using the Boyer Model to defend the activities associated with the Duquesne University School of Nursing Nurse-Managed Wellness Centers (DUSON NMWC) as being scholarly and appropriate for their faculty role. The following are some examples of how the Boyer Model was put into practice in the DUSON NMWC and used for evaluation.

Research

The DUSON NMWC is involved in a health literacy research program that involves teaching older adults to use the Internet to access health related information. Preliminary findings suggest that older adults are more interested in using the Internet for other uses such as communication with family via email, dating services, and playing cards.

Integration

In the DUSON NMWC, collaborations have been established with the Duquesne School of Pharmacy, Occupational Therapy Department, and Physical Therapy Department. Most recently, a collaboration began with the Computer Sciences Department to increase the use of computers and health literacy among older adults. The Generations for Healthy Living project provided a place for nursing, medicine, sociology, psychology, pharmacy, occupational therapy, physical therapy, and computer science to merge with the common goal of wellness. Both of these latter collaborations resulted in national presentations and publications are imminent.

Another example of integration as well as application is the "Walk & Win," a best practice program for the National Nursing Centers Consortium (NNCC), which was developed through a geriatric demonstration project involving six nursing centers, including the DUSON NMWC.

Application

The faculty members who staff the DUSON NMWC are the primary caregivers in these centers and therefore function as mentors and role models for the students assigned to the centers for clinical experiences. These faculty are also active participants in the NNCC, the American Academy of Nurse Practitioners, and special interest groups on nursing centers. They serve on a statewide health department task force to prevent fetal alcohol spectrum disorder. These are all examples of the scholarship of application. The conceptual framework of the Duquesne University School of Nursing is the *American Association of Critical Care Nurses (AACCN) Synergy Model for Patient Care* (AACN, n.d.). This model, which was originally created for an acute care environment, was applied to the DUSON's community-based curriculum and subsequently was applied to the wellness center model as another example of scholarship.

A final example of the scholarship of application involves grants. The distinction is often made between the value of program or project grants over research grants. The *RN+WIN Project* is the result of a program grant and is a direct application to solve a problem, which was how to sustain the DUSON NMWC and provide wellness activities for a larger population. This project involves the use of retired nurses who not only work with clients but also serve as mentors for students.

Teaching

The mission of the DUSON NMWC is to provide wellness-oriented health care services to vulnerable populations. However, a primary goal is to provide nursing and health science students with community-based, cross-cultural health care experiences. Students are routinely assigned to the NMWC. Some of the assignments facilitated by the faculty who manage the wellness centers are home safety assessments and follow-up, wellness screenings, complete health histories and physical exams, developmental assessments, and teaching projects. An innovative learning activity is a critical thinking case study approach for senior students. In this assignment, the students use the Synergy Model to assess characteristics of groups of patients who have chronic deviations from health. The objectives include internalizing behaviors of caring practice, using research as a basis for nursing interventions in chronic care, and fostering patient education in chronic care. Learning from student feedback enriches teaching. Teaching evaluations are completed by peers and students. In addition, clients are encouraged to do satisfaction surveys.

Summary

Boyer argued that recognition needs to be given to all four types of scholarship; that is, that scholarship must be interpreted in a broader manner. Scholarship needs to include definable objectives and clear goals, adequate preparation and understanding of the research in the discipline, and methods appropriate to support the project. A strategic plan that is congruent with the mission statement of the academic institution, the School of Nursing, and the nurse-managed wellness center should be developed and should include the above activities to form the basis for evaluation. Does the work of nurse-managed wellness centers reflect scholarship? Absolutely, and it can be used to show evidence of scholarly work for promotion and tenure.

Resources

This web resource contains a paper, *Boyer's Model of Scholarship,* authored by Martha Nibert: http://www.webs1.uidaho.edu/mkyte/ui_strategic_plan_implementation/resources/Boyer %20module%20Pacific%20Crest%20recd%209.4.06.pdf

This web resources contains a PowerPoint presentation, *Ernest Boyer's Model of Scholarship: An Overview,* by Dr. Ken Hansen. http://academic.csupomona.edu/ccsl/Presentations/ ernestboyer.ppt

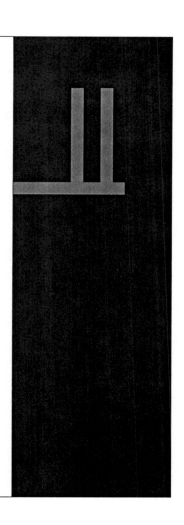

Development and Planning

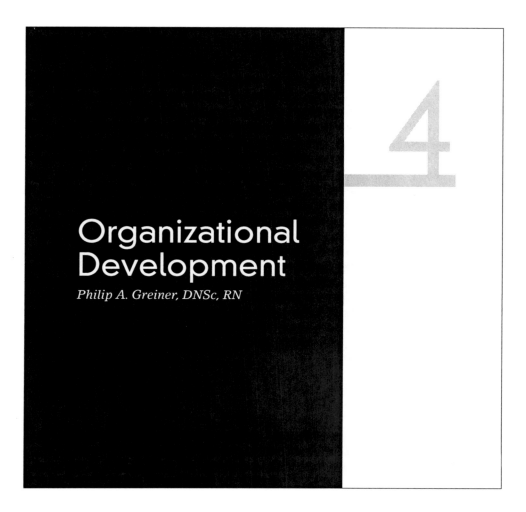

Organizational Development

Philip A. Greiner, DNSc, RN

The objectives of this chapter are to: identify the role of organizational mission in the decision-making process that leads to the formation of a wellness center, understand the complexity of planning and development needed for a successful wellness center, and create a checklist for planning and organizing a wellness center.

The chapter proposes a functional approach to developing a wellness center, outlines the development process, and suggests methods to operate the center. Throughout, examples are drawn from the experience of the writer with the Health Promotion Center (HPC) operated in Bridgeport, Connecticut, by the School of Nursing at Fairfield University in Fairfield, Connecticut, and from the experience of other directors of wellness centers.

Introduction

Nurse-managed wellness centers are most often linked to baccalaureate nursing programs within colleges or universities. Barger (1995) summarized the development of various nursing centers and indicated that schools of nursing have been engaged in the provision of health services for decades. Part of the motivation to begin a wellness center is to provide a place for student nurses to gain experience with community-based health promotion activities. But there are additional reasons why a wellness center in particular may be an excellent investment for a nursing program. Students can practice basic skills (taking blood pressures, performing finger sticks for blood sample collection), communication skills (gathering a brief health history, performing a structured interview, teaching about health concerns), beginning assessment skills (recognizing signs and symptoms typical of chronic disease states, observing deviations from normal anatomy and physiology), and more advanced skills (conducting a community assessment, setting priorities, translating health information into meaningful behaviors that people can follow). Through a wellness center, faculty members have the opportunity to develop and maintain connections with community agencies, gather data for research and publications, and create partnerships. Nursing programs and their parent institutions gain opportunities for service learning, outreach, and marketing. The ultimate goal is to create a site for student learning, faculty wellness practice and scholarship, and university visibility that is viable, sustainable, and valued in the community.

Corporate Status

As noted above, most nurse-managed wellness centers are operated by university schools of nursing and have advisory boards to guide their work. Those wellness centers have evolved from the mission of the school and/or university with which they are affiliated and operate as component parts of the parent universities rather than as free-standing corporations. This structure allows faculty to write grant proposals and obtain funding based on the non-profit status of the parent institution rather than going through the increasingly difficult process of applying for non-profit or corporate status for a new organization.

Another advantage of operating as a part of a university is that the university can function as the fiduciary agent in seeking funding, with the university managing the grant funds for an administrative fee. This university role as the fiduciary agent offers a distinct advantage if there are smaller community agency partners that may not have the infrastructure necessary to meet the requirements of granting agencies. By partnering with a wellness center affiliated with a university, a small community agency may qualify to obtain a grant and begin the process of building a funding track record.

Advisory or Governing Board

A wellness center should have a mechanism for gaining input from the community it serves. A board is one way to gain this input. The board may be an advisory board, if the center will operate under another organization, or a governing board, for independent organizations. If the wellness center is part of a larger organization, it is important that it adopt a structure to obtain community input and feedback that is compatible with that organization and with the community being served. For example, wellness centers that are housed in donated space may elect to have an advisory board that reflects the people being served and/or the agency donating the space. The advisory board gives the donating agency assurance that the wellness center is addressing population needs and may be a condition of occupancy of the donated space. Schools of nursing accredited by the Commission on Collegiate Nursing Education (CCNE) are required to seek input from their "communities of interest." A wellness center advisory board may represent such a community of interest, or the school of nursing may form a community board with representatives from the larger service community. In this latter case, a separate, specific wellness center advisory board may not be needed because input and feedback can be obtained from the community board.

For the HPC, a community advisory board was formed early in the development of the wellness center but was disbanded one year later because the members were part of several community groups and were unwilling to attend yet another meeting. The School of Nursing has a Partnership Council to gain feedback from the community and a School of Nursing Advisory Board for fund-raising purposes. Both groups receive periodic updates regarding the HPC and provide community input and feedback. In addition, faculty and staff from the HPC are involved in a number of community groups and boards, and there is a developing quality improvement program that includes patient and community surveys so that information flow back to the HPC is ensured. The bottom line is that a feedback process needs to be created that is appropriate to the wellness center's university, school or department, mission, and community.

Mission

One of the most important aspects of developing a wellness center is forging a mission for the center. The mission needs to be consistent with the mission of the parent institution, the mission of the school of nursing, and the identified needs within the community. The mission should be reflective of the goals of the wellness center in terms of the community, the students, the faculty, and the school. It should form a guide as decisions are made about the wellness center. The HPC mission statement follows as an example:

> The Health Promotion Center has as its mission the education of student nurses through service learning activities in the greater Bridgeport, CT, region. Activities are focused in two broad areas: the reduction of cardiovascular risk and the reduction of environmental hazards related to lead and other toxins. The HPC achieves these goals through partnerships with community organizations to provide health education, screening, and referrals.

The mission statement and accompanying vision, principles, and/or values should be short and clear and should convey the purpose of the wellness center to patients, staff, and funders. (See the profiles of example centers in Appendices A and B for sample mission statements.)

Getting Started

The decision to start a wellness center should be based on a sound understanding of the community, its assets and perceived needs, the populations to be served, available groups with whom to partner, and the resources available in that community. This information should lead to the identification of the specifics for the wellness center, including its location, mode of operation, staffing, and services to be provided.

The first action a faculty member should undertake in starting a wellness center is to make a complete assessment of the community. This assessment can be done at the beginning of the life of a wellness center and should be repeated on a regular basis as part of quality improvement. The assessment should take into account the availability of primary care providers, clinics, and other health-related services; vulnerable populations and their locations; public transportation routes; social service agencies and their services; and the basic demographics of the community and/or target neighborhoods. It is also advisable to talk with as many stakeholders as possible, such as people living in the community, service providers, religious leaders, and other key informants about existing health-related assets and perceived needs. With this information, decisions can be made regarding the best site for service provision and the services to provide.

Site Selection

One key assumption is that a university-related wellness center should usually be based in the community rather than on campus. Placing the wellness center in the community conveys a willingness on the part of the university to be present in the community and a commitment by the school to that community. The exception to this assumption is when the campus is embedded in the community itself or when the community members see the university as a resource within their community. Some wellness centers operate out of donated space in senior housing or other low-income housing. Others, such as the HPC, operate out of rented space within the area to be served. The HPC rents space in a Baptist Church. This church also rents space to other non-profit organizations and several other churches as a way of sustaining itself. In this way, Fairfield University also contributes to the viability of the community by paying rent.

How the wellness center is to operate is also important in choosing a location. Some wellness centers provide services at the center for a designated population. By locating within the communities, these centers are convenient to residents. For example, a Harrisburg, Pennsylvania based wellness center operating out of dedicated space in a senior housing unit allows residents to seek out the nurse when needed, yet also allows students to make "home visits" to residents on a regular basis. The HPC uses a different approach, a distributive model of public health, where services are delivered within partnering agencies. The HPC office is used more as a base of operations. Each approach is tailored to meet the needs of the designated population.

Financial Planning

Wellness centers can be very inexpensive to initiate and operate, which is one key reason to choose this approach over a primary care model. However, proper financial planning is key to the development, maintenance, and growth of a wellness center. An initial step in developing a financial plan for a wellness center is creating a list of assets and costs associated with its operation.

Assets: Assets include all of the items of value that make up the wellness center. This includes the time and expertise of faculty, staff, and students. The value of all donated time should be calculated at a reasonable rate for the region. For example, students are paid $15/hour for work done in the community for work-study jobs, which is consistent with what these students could earn in other jobs. Therefore, student service learning time is calculated at $15/hour times the number of hours and the number of students. Similarly, the faculty salary can be calculated for the number of course units taught over the semester at the HPC. These figures are important for calculating in-kind contributions for grants and other reporting requirements.

Assets include equipment, materials, and other items needed to conduct the activities of the wellness center. These items may be donated by the school, university, or community agencies. Examples of these assets include telephones and other office equipment, medical equipment such as stethoscopes, and educational materials. Much of the office furniture and equipment at the HPC are used materials from university storage, yet they are assets that allow the work of the center to take place. One caveat about accepting used equipment is that it must be in good operating condition and pose no threat of injury to students, staff, or patients.

Assets include all forms of income for the wellness center. Some centers charge for services. Charges must be set based on norms for the area and the population being served. Other centers have a donation container so that patients can donate if they so desire or offer services free of charge. The decision about charges should stem from the mission of the parent organization, take into account social justice issues, and reflect the relative value of the services to the community. The HPC does not charge a fee for services. Instead, support for the center comes from grant funding, sub-contracts, and donations. The decision not to charge for services was made after considerable discussion with administrators and faculty. Rendering free service in this manner places a considerable burden on faculty to secure grant funding to maintain HPC operations.

Regardless of the source of income, all funds flowing into the wellness center need to be accounted for and tracked. While support services are usually available through the parent organization, the center director should be familiar with financial management and budget development and monitoring. It is recommended that monthly financial reports be produced and reviewed to assure that funds are managed and reported accurately. It is also recommended that each funding source be given a separate account so that funds can be tracked according to grant requirements.

Costs: The cost of center operations needs to be reflected accurately for a variety of reasons. First, assuming that much of the center's income is through grant funding, the granting organization will need reporting on all expenditures.

Because wellness centers are linked to academic settings, faculty members tend to organize activities on an academic semester basis. Most other organizations track funding on a fiscal year (often July 1 – June 30) or grant year cycle (first day of the month grant was assigned – last day of the month preceding grant assignment). This is another reason for setting up each funding source as a separate account.

In addition to calculating annual costs, it is advantageous to also calculate a cost per person served. This cost calculation needs to be service-specific. For example, the cost for a blood pressure screening may be calculated on the number of students, hours of operation, and use of equipment such as alcohol wipes, blood pressure cuffs, and stethoscopes. Higher costs will be associated with screening activities involving a finger stick due to the use of more equipment, such as 2x2s, alcohol wipes, lancets, collection tubes, and screening cassettes. At the HPC, the equipment costs associated with cholesterol testing are $15/patient. The staffing costs are $7.50/patient. It is important to also demonstrate what the service would cost if an RN was hired to do the screening. In the southwestern Connecticut region, an RN would be paid $50/hour, screening four patients per hour at a per-patient staffing cost of $12.50.

While states differ in their requirements, most allow the use of Clinical Laboratory Improvement Amendments of 1988 (CLIA)-waived testing in the community (CDC, 2008). CLIA-waived tests include urine and/or blood testing for cholesterol, glucose, and Hemoglobin A1c, which must be conducted using CLIA-waived equipment. One focus for many wellness centers, including the HPC, is cardiovascular wellness. As a result, CLIA-waived Cholestex LDX machines were purchased with grant funds so that students could offer cholesterol and glucose testing with one finger stick. CLIA-waived equipment was obtained by donation for testing glucose and Hemoglobin A1c in the community. In order to use CLIA-waived equipment, wellness centers must apply to their State Department of Health for a CLIA waiver and pay the related fee.

The cost of equipment, office supplies, paper, photocopying, educational materials, space rental and utilities, telephone and Internet access, and staff all contribute to the overall cost of operations. While it may be difficult to anticipate all of the associated operating costs prior to opening, construction of an accurate budget depends on a credible attempt to capture these elements.

Value Added: Much of the value of having a wellness center is not directly evident. Administrators look at the cost of operations in relation to available funding. Faculty members look at the relevance of the clinical experiences to specific courses and/or course content. Students look at the types of skills acquired in relation to clinical aspirations and course outcomes. It may be more appropriate to look at the value added by having a wellness center.

Value-added is defined by Merriam-Webster (2008) as something added to a product that increases its value or worth. If the product of nursing education is a well-educated, socially just nurse, then the task is to identify the value-added components of having a wellness center as part of the experience for students and faculty. Since service learning is an integral part of nursing education, any estimation of the value added by a wellness center must include the benefit to society in general and the population served in particular. One example is the fact that students working in centers that serve underserved communities have a great opportunity for cultural competency training and experience in working with poor and minority populations.

Staffing

Staffing of wellness centers varies according to a variety of factors, the most important of which is funding. It is not uncommon for wellness centers to develop using faculty time and effort as the basis for staffing. This time and effort may come from course time (if the wellness center activities are integrated into specific courses), released time, or faculty overload. The amount of time and effort dedicated to wellness center operations is frequently not sufficient for the work required. It is recommended that, to help in documenting the time and effort needed by the center, time be recorded for the first few years of operations much the way lawyers record their time and effort — in 15-minute time blocks. For example, if the Director spent 30 minutes arranging for screening activities during a given day, those 30 minutes are recorded along with the activity into a log. This log may be a physical book or a record in an Excel spreadsheet (so that hours may be easily added).

With external funding, full- or part-time staff can be added to the wellness center. Adding positions needs to be done with input from Human Resources and the Dean of the School. Costs include salary, benefits, and FICA. These costs must be calculated at the rates set for the parent university. In all cases, new positions need to have job descriptions that outline the work and justify the pay scale. The wellness center also needs policies developed for the interface of staff and faculty, staff and students, and staff and community agencies; excused and unexcused absences; and vacation and sick time; as well as probation and evaluation. Human Resources specialists are vital to making sure that all aspects are covered.

Staffing may include students, work study, community volunteers, and VISTA volunteers. Each of these groups may require scheduling and documentation of time and effort for internal and external reporting. If these positions are grant funded, tracking of budget expenditures may also fall to the wellness center director. The wellness center should have an organizational chart showing a direct link within the school or department. When staff are added at the wellness center, the organizational chart should be revised to define lines of reporting and communication.

Hours of Operation

Part of the decision-making process includes determining when the wellness center will be open. Wellness centers do not need to be open 24/7 or have 24/7 coverage. If staffing falls solely on faculty, center hours may vary each semester. If the center has external funding, there may be requirements in the funding that dictate a minimum of hours that the center needs to be open. The hours of operation relate directly to the model of operation for the center. For instance, a wellness center in low-income housing may keep regular hours, such as Monday through Wednesday from 10 a.m. to 2 p.m., that are determined with input from the advisory board or housing tenants' council. The HPC does not keep regular hours of operation because of the distributive approach used, where agencies schedule HPC activities to come to their facilities. All business is conducted by initial telephone and e-mail contact.

In any case, the wellness center needs to have a dedicated telephone number and e-mail address so that community members can reach the center director and/or staff. It is key that messages be responded to in a timely manner. The center director may elect to use a cell phone instead of a landline, particularly if fax services are not needed. Also, the possibility of getting a university-sourced cell phone can be explored. Organizations that have many cell phones where the majority of calls are made within the provider network may have thousands of unused minutes available for wellness center use. Similarly, obtaining computer and Internet access through university sources may be possible. The HPC is on the university computer replacement list, so a new and upgraded computer is provided every three to four years. Internet access is provided by the church as part of the rental fee.

Business Plan

Every wellness center should have a business plan that is revised every year. If the university business office does not provide such support, the U. S. Small Business Administration provides web-based tools to develop a business plan at http://www.sba.gov/smallbusinessplanner/plan/writeabusinessplan/index. html. In using this resource, a wellness center can elect to use only the pieces that apply to its services. A business plan allows non-nurses, such as administrators in the university, to assess the center's planning and determine where organizational supports can be made available. It can also be useful in applying for grant funding.

Conclusion

The chances of a wellness center's survival increase if careful thought is given initially to all aspects of center development. For many nurses, clinical skills will not be applicable to what is essentially a business venture. Ask for assistance in developing this venture. Use resources readily available within your university. Work with a community partner to gain expertise that may not be available in-house. Ask another wellness center administrator for guidance. Plan for success!

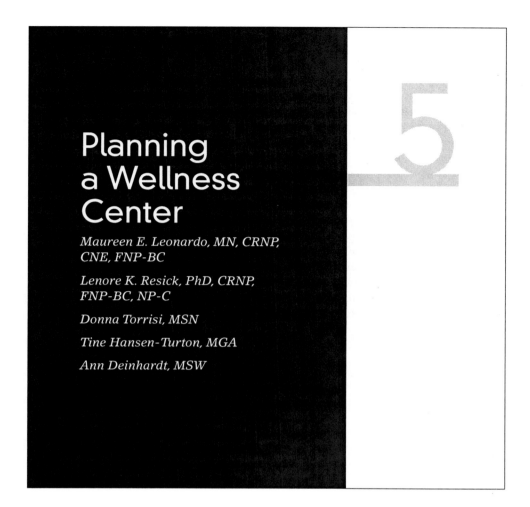

Planning a Wellness Center

Maureen E. Leonardo, MN, CRNP, CNE, FNP-BC

Lenore K. Resick, PhD, CRNP, FNP-BC, NP-C

Donna Torrisi, MSN

Tine Hansen-Turton, MGA

Ann Deinhardt, MSW

Introduction

Planning a wellness center is much the same as planning a small business. The process includes a community assessment, a feasibility study, a business plan, a strategic plan, a financial plan that includes start-up costs, a sustainability plan, and an evaluation plan. Issues regarding institutional, political, business, legal, regulatory, policy, and safety concerns must be considered in the planning process. The objective of this chapter is to discuss points to consider in planning a wellness center. This chapter will focus specifically on the community needs assessment, planning a center, and academic or parent organization buy-in.

Community and Needs Assessments

Most simplistically, a community is an entity made up of people, a place, and social systems. It may include a large area such as a city, town, or region, or it may be a local site such as an apartment complex or a place of employment. Through community assessment, someone planning a wellness center is able to determine how the community influences the health of its residents. Community assessment can be used to ascertain the health status, resources, and needs of groups of individuals. A community assessment should always be done, although the process may vary according to the community of interest. Since a community assessment is not done in a vacuum, planners may already be familiar with some aspects of the community by virtue of their involvement in the community. This information may guide how the assessment is conducted.

The focus of the needs assessment should be on the community's strengths and existing resources. Any community organizations that have similar interests and that may be potential collaborators or competitors should be identified and studied. This type of review can reduce the chance of duplication of services and lead to a comprehensive array of services through collaboration and resource sharing. Other benefits of collaboration or affiliation may be the promotion of commitment to community health improvement efforts, the activation of citizens to participate in health decision-making, and the promotion of a shared vision regarding community health goals and outcomes (Clemen-Stone, McGuire, & Eigsti, 2002).

Community Assessment

There are many methods that can be used to conduct a community assessment, which will look for both assets and needs. Some of these methods used are:

- *Windshield survey,* a "motorized equivalent of a simple head-to-toe assessment" (Hunt, 2009, p. 146). This survey is done by observing the community of interest on a drive through the community (a foot walk for a smaller community). Planners should use their powers of observation to conduct a general assessment using all five senses. This will provide information about the way people live, where they live, housing, health status, and so forth.
- *Secondary data collection* utilizing records, documents, and other resources. Examples of these are the demographic data and ethnicity, morbidity, and mortality statistics (vital statistics) from the local health department and school health records.
- *Formal surveys* provided to a sample of the targeted population. These may entail significant expense and typically do not have a good rate of return.
- *Informant interviews* involving community residents who are key informants or just members of the general public. Key informants are individuals who are influential in the community. Sometimes these individuals have formal positions, such as positions in government, business, or religion. Others have informal positions but are influential nonetheless. These individuals may also be known as gatekeepers.
- *Participant observation* in which formal and informal communities activities are observed. Some formal activities may be local government meetings, tenant council meetings, or organization meetings. Informal activities may include gatherings at a local coffee shop, barbershop, or hair salon, or house meetings. This method can be very effective in determining values, norms, and concerns of a community.

Needs Assessment

The needs assessment is actually a part of the community assessment. This should also be an ongoing assessment to meet the possible changing needs of the community being served once the wellness center is established. (See Appendix D-5 for an example of a tool that can be used as part of a needs assessment.)

Community Needs: Once the stakeholders and the community leaders are determined, some questions that should be considered are:

- What is the most effective way for entry into the community?
- Who are the gatekeepers? A gatekeeper is a term used to refer to a person or persons who control the flow of information. These are the individuals who allow information to pass through them to be disseminated to the public. A gatekeeper decides what information the public should receive and what information should be accepted, rejected, or kept from public consumption. They are an invaluable source of information about the community and an invaluable resource to gather information about the target community.
- Who are the official and unofficial community leaders?

The answers to these questions will provide information for the several methods that can be used to conduct a needs assessment (or any data collection) that includes all the stakeholders. These may include participant observation, informant interviews, and focus groups. Focus groups are a powerful means to get new ideas such as the community's ideas about wellness and how it perceives its needs, and to evaluate services once the wellness center is established. McNamara (n.d.) provides excellent information on the basics of conducting focus groups at: http://www.managementhelp.org/evaluatn/focusgrp.htm.

By using the community's perspective, a wellness center can be established that is community-based and community-focused. The services that will be provided are based on those identified as needed by the community that is being served. It is important to consider services that augment existing services but do not duplicate them.

Academic or Partnering Institution Needs: If the wellness center is affiliated with a larger parent institution such as a school of nursing that is part of a university, the needs of the academic or partnering institution should also be considered as they are also stakeholders. The wellness center is a bridge between theory and practice, integrating the scholarship of research, teaching, and practice, and operationalizing the mission statement of the institution.

Feasibility Study

An important component of the assessment process is a feasibility study. A feasibility study is an assessment of what will be offered, who it will be offered to and how many, and who or what will be the competition or partners. The feasibility study also asks the question, "Is there a fit between the demand and the services being offered?" In summary, a feasibility study determines the current market, the costs, the existence of duplicate services, and the probability of the success of the wellness center. This information can be used to determine the purpose and scope of practice.

Planning the Wellness Center

Once the assessment process is completed, the planning process begins. Wellness centers are part of a continuum of health care services and can be free standing or affiliated with larger institutions. The community assessment is used to help determine the purpose of the wellness center and a realistic scope of practice. A number of other items need to be taken into consideration when determining the scope of practice in addition to the perceived needs of the community. In the case of a center that is affiliated with a university, these include the resources of the university and the university mission statement, as well as possible funding sources.

Purpose and Scope of Practice

In conducting the initial community assessment, there are some specific questions to ask to determine the focus and population of the wellness center. Focus on the areas where you have a distinct advantage. Identify the problem in your target market for which your service or product provides a solution. Some of the questions to ask include:

- Will the wellness center direct care to a specific health need (diabetes, HIV) or to a particular age group (young families, older adults), gender, or socioeconomic population (low income)? What are the demographics and ethnicity of the community?
- What are the morbidity and mortality rates of the community? How do these statistics compare to the region, state, and national statistics? (morbidity and mortality statistics of the local health department)
- Who are the obvious stakeholders? Who are the not-so-obvious stakeholders? (stakeholders and community leaders)
- What are the resources and barriers of both the community and the parent organization?

If the wellness center is affiliated with a larger parent institution, such as a school of nursing that is part of a university, the mission statement of the institution, must be taken into consideration. Does the mission statement fit with the goals and objectives of a wellness center? The mission statement of the institution and school will determine administrative and faculty "buy-in." Another consideration is the guiding framework or nursing theory supported by the school of nursing's curricula. The wellness center needs to support the school's framework. Some preliminary questions for nursing faculty to ask include:

- What services can be offered?
- How much time will this take? Can the time commitment be managed? Will release time be available?

- Is there a faculty practice plan in place?
- Does the academic institution recognize the scholarship of application?
- Who are the stakeholders?
- What will this cost?
- How will income be generated? Will income be generated?
- Is the parent organization willing to assist in efforts toward sustainability?
- Who are the champions to keep the wellness center going?

A Written Plan

A written guide containing a strategic plan, a business plan, and financial plan is just as essential to planning a small wellness center as it is to a large business venture.

Strategic Plan: An organization that is planning to develop a wellness center should first create a comprehensive, written strategic plan that covers a three- to five-year period and includes a business plan and a long-range financial plan. An internal assessment should be done as part of the planning process that includes a SWOT (Strengths, Weaknesses, Opportunities, and Threats) analysis and considers the organization's resources as well as its limitations. The strategic plan contains the mission and vision statement of the wellness center. The mission and vision statements determine the long-term and short-term goals, the priorities, and the outcomes to be accomplished by the wellness center. The strategic plan also details the range of services that will be provided, either directly or indirectly, and the number of practitioners and other staff needed to operate, as well as their required credentials. The center's need for volunteers and use of students should also be considered. The mechanisms for including the community in the planning and management of the center and its services should be part of the plan, as should the center's plan for participating in the community and local, state, and national networks.

A strategic planning process should be completed at least once every three to five years. Each year, annual plans should be developed that support the goals of the strategic plan and allow for changes in strategies as the environment and internal processes of the wellness center change. (See Appendix D-5 for three examples of strategic plans.)

Business and Financial Planning: Issues to be addressed in business planning include marketing, partnership building (e.g., a community board and/or collaborators), financial planning, personnel needs, and budgets, as well as a time line and hours of operation. Planning also includes record keeping, the electronic data management system to be used, risk management issues, workplace safety, and quality assurance measures. Many resources are available through the United States Government Small Business Administration to help in business planning. The web site of the U.S. Government Small Business Administration, http://www.sba.gov/smallbusinessplanner/plan/writeabusinessplan/index.html, provides forms and information on how to write a complete business plan. In addition to forms, the website also offers a number of free online courses related to starting a business or business planning.

Financial planning includes start-up costs and sustainability. Financial planning for setting up a wellness center is often not as difficult as financial planning for the sustainability of a primary care health center since many services provided by wellness centers are not directly reimbursable by third-party payers. The financial plan addresses whether clients will be charged a fee for services. Consideration in planning is directly related to the availability of grants, reimbursement, donations, and profit-generating collaborative agreements. Financial planning includes start-up costs, daily operating costs, overhead, equipment, supplies, capital expenses, salary, support staff, insurance, and contracts. Funding will be covered in another chapter.

Budget: Creating and following a budget is essential to the survival of a wellness center. The annual budget should reflect the goals of the center and should be dynamic so that it can be adjusted to reflect changes in the business environment. The budget should take into consideration funding anticipated during the year, the fixed and incremental costs of operation, and potentially changing costs and conditions. It must consider the personnel necessary to accomplish long-term and short-term goals and the workloads to be carried by staff members. The development of the annual budget should include a review of the long-range financial plan that is part of the strategic plan. The governing Board in independent organizations and the university in those associated with schools of nursing should approve the annual budget before the beginning of each fiscal year.

The annual budget includes revenues, operating expenses including state and federal taxes, and cash flow projections. Revenues are the funds that the organization has and plans to acquire to pay the bills. Operating expenses include rent, insurance, payroll costs, taxes, supplies, building maintenance, interests on loans, and overhead. The budget will help forecast cash needs of the business and control expenditures. The management and the Board should review fiscal statements no less than quarterly to examine the relationship of the budget to actual expenditures and revenues and to examine issues of fiscal policies and procedures.

Policies and Procedures

Policies and procedures guide the work of the wellness center and promote quality of services, consistency of performance, safety, sound business practices, and communication of standards and expectations throughout the organization. They are essential for providing clear guidelines and rationale for staff practice and behaviors. Wellness center policies and procedures should be written and should reflect the center's mission, vision, and goals. Involving staff in the development of policies and procedures, whenever practical and appropriate, promotes staff engagement and helps to ensure that they are comprehensive and relevant to staff practice.

For centers associated with universities, policies are likely to be adopted from the school. For independent organizations, the Board should approve center policies. Organizational and Service procedures are developed by the center to detail how the policies will be implemented. (See Appendix D-5 for a sample Table of Contents for a Policy and Procedure Manual.)

Local, State, and Federal Regulations: When developing policies and procedures, the wellness center should be aware of all local, state, federal, and contractual regulations that impact on the operations of the center. State laws govern the scope of practice, prescriptive authority and collaboration require-ments for nurse-managed wellness centers, while state and federal laws address the care of patients covered by Medical Assistance and Medicare. Governance of Nurse Practitioner practice varies by state and may involve oversight by the State Board of Nursing or joint oversight with the State Board of Medicine. Organizations should stay current on state legislation and be involved in coali-tions and task forces that are impacting the rules and regulations that govern nursing practice and health centers.

Organizational Policies and Procedures

Organizational policies outline the broad management and administrative func-tions of the health center, delineate the broad responsibilities of staff members, establish such basic requirements as the code of ethics and patient rights, and require the maintenance of quality services. These and personnel policies are generally adopted from the university or approved by the Board.

Organizational procedures spell out how the broad policies will be imple-mented and include: risk management procedures, personnel procedures, financial procedures, and other administrative procedures that include those that guide the management of information and adherence to HIPAA require-ments, as well as those that establish processes for the establishment of written collaboration agreements, research, staff travel, public relations and relations with the media, staff development and training, and fundraising.

Risk Management Procedures: Wellness centers should have a risk management plan that assures that required codes are followed, property is well-maintained and inspected regularly, safety activities and safety-related trainings are carried out, adequate insurances are carried, and quality improve-ment information is used to help reduce organization liability.

Facilities in which wellness centers are located should meet all local, state, and licensing codes, as well as Section 504 of the Rehabilitation Act of 1973 and the Americans with Disabilities Act (ADA). Certificates that indicate codes are met and inspections such as those by the Fire Department should be kept on file. Facilities should be inspected regularly to assure that they are clean, well-maintained, and friendly and welcoming for consumers. Emergency kits and other equipment should be part of the inspections to assure that they are fully stocked with in-date supplies. Also, the requirements of the Occupational Safety & Health Administration (OSHA) need to be followed regarding protec-tion of employees from the possibility of exposure to blood or other potentially infectious materials. Employees must be offered required vaccinations and pro-cedures must be implemented to minimize or eliminate employee exposure to bloodborne and airborne pathogens. The risk management plan should outline the annual conduction of fire drills, mock codes, and staff training in such areas as infection control and crisis management, as well as field safety for staff who work in the community. All staff need to be trained in risk management proce-dures, since they are the first line of defense in identifying problems that could become liabilities for the organization.

Adequate insurance coverage is essential for any kind of health services. The types of coverage that must be carried are: comprehensive general liability insurance for the facility and the organization; professional liability, or malpractice, insurance for the health care providers; and officers' and directors' liability insurance if there is a governing board. Familiarity and compliance with practice protocols and guidelines, as well as state laws, is one way of preventing lawsuits.

Whether the nurse-managed health center is affiliated with a hospital or university will be one factor in determining the type of malpractice coverage that should be obtained for the nursing professionals employed by the health center. According to Buppert (2004), it is recommended that practitioners have "occurrence" insurance, which covers any incident while the health professional is insured. A "claims made" insurance policy only covers the person when the insurance policy is active, regardless of when the incident occurred. "Tail coverage" can be purchased for a period of time equivalent to the state's statute of limitations for that act of malpractice (Esposito, 2000). Other considerations are the amount of the coverage and the specific acts that are covered by the insurance.

Personnel Policies and Procedures: It is helpful to have someone available to the organization that has personnel management expertise. Personnel policies may come from the university or may be approved by the board. The personnel policies should be published in a manual that is distributed to all employees, with signatures regarding their receipt of the manual and any updates/changes. These policies and their accompanying procedures will help the wellness center manage its employees and govern its employment practices in conformity with applicable laws and regulations, including but not limited to the Civil Rights Act of 1964, the Fair Labor Standards Act (as amended by the Equal Pay Act and the Age Discrimination in Employment Act), the Occupational Safety and Health Act, the Americans with Disabilities Act, the National Labor Relations Act, the Family and Medical Leave Act, and the Rehabilitation Act of 1973, as well as applicable state and local laws. Legal counsel should be consulted when personnel policies are developed or revised and when necessary to assure the agency's conformity to legal requirements.

The organization should determine, through the planning and budgeting process, the appropriate number, qualifications, and credential requirements of the staff needed to carry out day-to-day operations and achieve the goals and objectives of the wellness center. A written position classification structure with pay ranges should be developed and used for all positions. A benefits package should also be defined and employees kept informed of any changes in it. The organization should carry workers' compensation insurance, payroll insurance, and health insurance for employees in accordance with state laws and must contribute to FICA for all personnel. It should be determined and stated in policy which staff are eligible for medical insurance, unemployment benefits, tax-deferred accounts, and paid vacation.

Job descriptions that define the experience and qualifications required for the position and specify the duties and responsibilities and outcomes-oriented performance expectations, as well as credentials and other requirements necessary to fulfill the responsibilities of the job, should be maintained for all positions. (See Appendix D-5 for sample job descriptions.) Care must be taken to assure that positions are properly classified according to Federal Wage and Hour Regulations. Procedures for recruitment and hiring should be followed to eliminate, to the degree possible, any discrimination. The procedures of an established organization and such resources as the Internal Revenue Service's website, which provides a helpful tax guide for employers, should be used when developing hiring procedures. Legal counsel should be consulted to assure that all requirements are met. Staffing and hiring should be reviewed regularly to assure that the organization is adhering to the civil rights requirements of any public funders.

Staff development procedures should be followed that assure that all personnel receive a full orientation to the organization, its policies and procedures, and the specifics of their position. These procedures should also specify ongoing training requirements and requirements for annual employee performance review. In order to hold personnel accountable for their responsibilities, the competence of each employee to fulfill the work responsibilities described in the job description should be assessed through performance reviews conducted at the end of the probation period and annually. Employees perform best when they have the tools they need to do their work, receive regular feedback from their supervisor, and are engaged in their work. Employees are entitled to regular feedback from their supervisor. This should not be limited to the formal annual review but should occur frequently and include concrete examples of how successful the employee is in meeting tasks described in their job description.

Financial Procedures: Financial procedures should be in place to provide reasonable assurance regarding the efficiency of operations, reliability of financial reporting, and compliance with applicable laws and regulations. These should include:

- Procedures for budget development, monitoring, variance analysis, and audit;
- Procedures requiring an accrual method of accounting and prompt and accurate recording of revenues and expenses;
- Separation of accounting duties to the extent possible and other controls;
- Procedures for the review and approval of payroll expenditures, time and overtime records, and written authorization for payroll changes;
- Purchasing procedures, including authorization levels for expenditures;
- Additional procedures, such as bank reconciliations, accounts receivable reconciliation, and fee and reimbursement collection.

HIPAA and Confidentiality: Administrative policies and procedures must address the need for confidentiality regarding patient information. In many cases, these must take into consideration the Health Insurance Portability and Accountability Act of 1996 (HIPAA), which was designed to protect health coverage for workers and their families when they change or lose their jobs, assure the privacy of medical information, and standardize electronic data interchange. The HIPAA Standards for Privacy of Individually Identifiable Health Information are a comprehensive set of federal rules aimed at providing confidentiality protection to nearly all medical records and other individually identifiable health information and call for unique health identifiers for individuals, employers, health plans, and health care providers. Health care organizations, health plans, health care clearinghouses, and health care providers need to be familiar with HIPAA requirements and comply with them or face civil and criminal penalties. Many wellness centers will not need to be HIPAA compliant since they do not receive reimbursement for their services. Although these centers may not have a HIPAA statement, it is essential that they have and enforce confidentiality procedures.

Service Procedures

Services in the wellness center, including support services, should have procedures to guide the staff in the performance of their responsibilities. These procedures should be detailed and developed and updated in accordance with good practice and the requirements of the regulators and funding sources of the services. The procedures should be used in the orientation and training of staff and should be formally reviewed by staff and management at least once every two years. Procedures should detail how each service is provided; how referrals are made and tracked; the handling of emergencies; reporting of incidents and accidents, reportable illnesses and conditions, and child abuse and neglect; and such issues as patient grievances, working with handicapped patients, cultural competence, and hazardous waste disposal.

Summary

Planning a wellness center is much the same as planning any small business. Community involvement and identification of resources and needs from all stakeholders are essential components in the planning process. Planning involves building upon the identified resources and developing a strong infrastructure toward a win-win situation for all involved.

Resources

Web site of the US Government Small Business Association that provides forms and information on how to write a complete business plan: http://www.sba.gov/smallbusiness planner/plan/writeabusinessplan/index.html

Web site from the US Government Small Business Association for registration for the online course on how to write a business plan: http://app1.sba.gov/sbtn/registration/index.cfm?CourseId=27

Information on the basics of conducting focus groups: http://www.managementhelp.org/evaluatn/focusgrp.htm

Web resource on the use of windshield surveys for the purpose of health changes: http://www.cdc.gov/dhdsp/library/seh_handbook/chapter_five.htm

Torrisi, D. L., & Hansen-Turton, T. (2005). Introduction in *Community and Nurse-Managed Health Centers: Getting Them Started and Keeping Them Going*. New York: Springer Publishing Company.

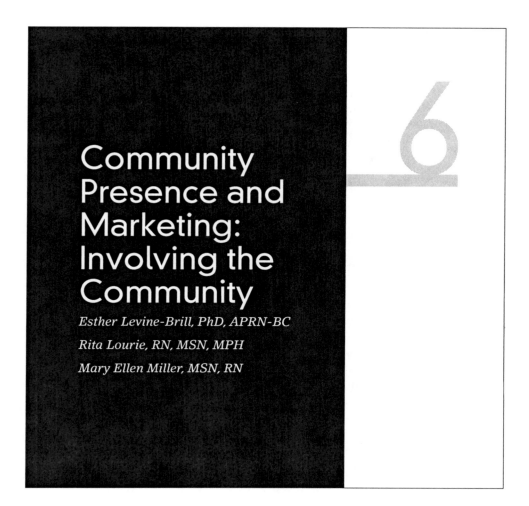

Community Presence and Marketing: Involving the Community

Esther Levine-Brill, PhD, APRN-BC

Rita Lourie, RN, MSN, MPH

Mary Ellen Miller, MSN, RN

Building Bridges

Community involvement is imperative for the success of a Wellness Center and usually precedes the establishment of a Wellness or Nursing Center. Some Schools of Nursing have been working in the community for years; other times a community agency has approached the School of Nursing or a nursing organization to provide needed services. There is no clear blueprint for developing partnerships in the community to be served, so nursing center teams are encouraged to experiment by expanding the development team in meaningful ways and avoid the paralysis that can be caused by uncertainty about what services will work best for the community.

One suggestion for attaining community buy-in involves holding focus groups. One center held focus groups for specific segments of the population: expectant parents, pre-school parents, Home and School/PTA parents, and Senior Citizens. At the same time, the nursing center team was making one-on-one appointments with community leaders, health agency directors, and so forth, to explain the vision of the center and elicit hopes, wishes, and dreams, as well as frustrations of the community agencies, with the goal of making their participation with the nursing center into a win-win situation. Each team representative had an "elevator speech" which described the nursing center in the time it would take an elevator to go from the first floor to the top and prepared for each visit with an explanation of how the center could enhance the services provided by the particular community agency and how the skills and services of the agency or person could enhance the nursing center. Other nursing center groups have done windshield surveys or community assessments to identify what was lacking in the area and then to develop a plan to see if this was something the community would welcome.

Stakeholders

Having community members be a part of the center by serving on the board of directors or advisory board is a major way of building bridges with the community and maintaining and sustaining community involvement (Rothman, Lourie, Gass, & Dyer, 2000). The key players or stakeholders may appear to be self evident, but there are a number of entities in the community who should be considered:

Politicians: Depending upon the legislative structure of the community, these might include City Council members, Township officials, and legislative aides of area congressmen or senators in their local offices. Their buy-in is important for establishing a presence in the community and can help with real estate issues, potential funding opportunities, and further on down the road, policy issues.

Strategic Planners: These people might be found on other boards as government relations officers, faculty in urban studies departments, or authorities in public policy. This member of a nursing center board can provide consultation around strategic planning, organizational development, communications, and community and governmental relations.

Marketing/Public Relations: Representatives from local radio, local TV, public relations firms, and local newspapers can be invited to join the board. This board member can help craft the center's message, help plan strategies for message dissemination, and might help to gauge the affect of any campaign.

Financial Experts: An accountant, a representative from a civic-minded bank, or a financial planner can be a very important person on the board. The resources available from a parent institution will determine how involved this person will be. Some non-profits utilize this person as the Treasurer of the board who can track the finances of the organization.

Community Members: These board members should be chosen from those who have voiced interest in the center and active members of the community, such as Home and School/PTA or tenant council officers or religious leaders. It can be advantageous to have a youth representative and a prominent senior citizen, as well. These board members can help in identifying ongoing areas of community need and communicating the center's activities to community members.

Social Service Agencies: Collaborative relationships can be developed with other agencies dealing with health, education, and wellness including Head Starts, schools, youth agencies, library administration, Health Department representatives, United Way, and so forth.

Safety Officers: Representatives of police, fire, and university security or other agencies to which the center might turn in time of increased need are also good possibilities for board membership.

Students: Undergraduate and graduate students from various disciplines can be engaged in all aspects of nursing center activities. As board members, they can provide their impressions of community needs and augment an interdisciplinary team.

Maintaining the Bridges

Community involvement needs to be carefully cultivated and nurtured to be sustained. The leadership of the nursing center should work on promoting a democratic environment with goals of shared power and decision-making. The mission of the wellness center might include language directed towards goals of community capacity building and sustainability beyond the end of any specific project or program.

There are several techniques or mechanisms that can be employed at meetings to keep community members involved:

Hold Regular Meetings and Foster Relationships: Some centers have monthly meetings; others meet seasonally with four meetings a year. The first and best option for meeting is face-to-face meetings held in a local community center, church, school, or restaurant. Refreshments, transportation, and parking should be taken into consideration in choosing the location. Start each such meeting with introductions of the participants and be sure to have nameplates on the table to identify members by name and affiliation. Some groups take advantage of free conferencing calls arranged through various Web sites found by searching "free conference calling." Remote areas, such as rural Alaska where there are no landlines, rely on satellite transmissions that require the use of narrow bandwidth telecommunications and information technology. It is a good idea to follow up each meeting with phone calls to key players thanking them for their input and possibly reminding them of work that remains to be done for the group.

Structure Agendas for Interest: Every meeting should be action-oriented where opinions are garnered and considered. Nothing is more boring than a meeting built entirely on reports. An initial meeting might consider a "value clarification exercise," where everyone contributes a laundry list of important issues in the community. These issues are printed on large pieces of paper and taped to the wall. Each member has three Post-Its with the numbers 1, 2, or 3 written on them. Then the board members and staff place the Post-Its on the issue sheets so they can be added up to determine the order of priority; the issue with the most 1's is considered the first priority.

Employ Community Members: Whenever possible, members of the community being served should be hired as outreach workers or even as consultants on grants. One center noted that "Community consultants review all our research, help us refine the methods, help get rid of our academic research language, and help interpret our results. Their input has lead to substantial changes in research design."

An Easy WIN: The first activity, project, or program should be short-term, involving the maximum number of members and member organizations possible. A health fair is often considered for the first initiative with active brainstorming, roles for all—including students—and an evaluation mechanism in place for reporting and redesigning subsequent activities.

Pay Back: Just as the nursing center leadership wants community members and agencies involved in the center, they are likely to expect the center leaders to become involved in their organizations. Participation in the community can only lead to a stronger safety net and improved programs for the population the nursing center is designed to serve.

Mending Bridges

Every group experiences some problems or misunderstandings. As in any relationship, it is worthwhile to confront the problem head-on before it festers and threatens to destroy the relationships that have been so carefully tended. Taking responsibility for the problem is always a wise step (even if you are certain it was not your fault). "I heard there's a problem. I want to apologize for anything I or a member of my staff did or said to cause you any discomfort," "Tell me what happened and let's see what we can do to rectify the situation."

Celebrate Successes

Celebrate every success—with food, prizes, medals, awards, or award certificates. Celebrate birthdays, births, marriages, graduations, new additions, and retirements. Create cards with your logo or a picture of the nursing center and send it to the center's community partners to continually thank them for their involvement or to congratulate them on a success of their own.

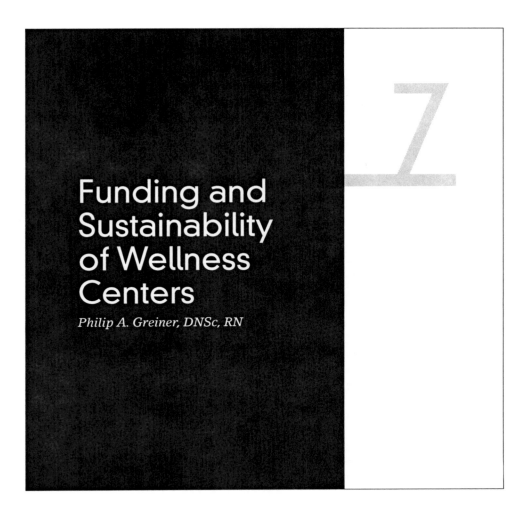

Funding and Sustainability of Wellness Centers

Philip A. Greiner, DNSc, RN

Introduction

The terms funding and sustainability represent separate but related concepts. The purpose of this chapter is to differentiate the two concepts, identify possible funding sources, and encourage planning for sustainability. Examples will be used to highlight the process developed at the Health Promotion Center (HPC), Fairfield University School of Nursing's wellness center located in Bridgeport, CT.

Unlike nursing centers with a primary care focus, wellness centers have not substantially benefited from federal funding support. An earlier review of nursing centers by Barger (1995) points out that when start-up funding ended, many of the federally funded nursing centers were unable to sustain themselves. Wellness centers may not have the overhead costs that primary care centers have, but the issues of sources of funding and sustainability remain.

Funding

Many wellness centers begin on a shoestring budget. Often, the Dean of the school of nursing makes a limited amount of funding available for initial start-up in donated space. While this approach may get the center off the ground, funding is usually short-term and the donated space may not be adequate for the services provided as the center develops. Initial funding for some wellness centers has come from university budget surpluses, but this may be a thing of the past with current funding shortfalls. Again, this approach is short-term. It is recommended that the program plan and related funding be well planned and considered.

Fee-for-Service

It is possible to charge a fee for the services provided through a wellness center. In particular, the cost of screening activities and related education can have a cost attached to them. This fee may be paid by the patient directly or may be paid by a community organization. Some insurance providers may be willing to contract to pay for screening activities on a per-person basis. In general, however, it is difficult to use fee-for-service as the basis of wellness center activities.

Grants

Grants are a common source of funding for wellness center activities. The key is to apply for grant funding that fits the mission of the wellness center, rather than having the wellness center activities driven by available grant funding. Funding organizations include local and regional foundations, state and federal grants administered through regional organizations, and larger foundations and federal grants. Most universities have an office of grant management or similar organizational structure to assist faculty in finding and submitting grant applications. These grants personnel can be very helpful in identifying granting organizations that fit the goals and mission of the wellness center.

Some larger granting organizations will provide project funding for up to three years, while small grants may be available for shorter time frames. For example, Area Agencies on Aging have Older American's Act funding to support health promotion and medication management activities for older adults. These grants are for one year, but grant proposals can be submitted each year.

Another source of small grants is from family foundations. These family foundations are often small with targeted areas of giving. However, sometimes family foundations reach the end of their fiscal year with funds left that need to be distributed. The foundation relations person within the university may know of family foundations with an affinity for your university or a focus in the area of health services. By sending these contacts information about your wellness center, the foundation relations person may find funding that needs to be spent.

Grants have specific management and reporting requirements that add to the work of the wellness center director. Reporting can range from quarterly to annual, and management may require specific documentation of faculty and student time in service provision. Once the wellness center has an established record managing grants, it may be easier to receive additional grant funding. Request for Proposal (RFP) requirements should be looked at closely, keeping in mind that small grant applications and management can be as demanding as those for larger grants. The director should seek assistance in developing skill in reviewing RFPs so that s/he can quickly decide if there is a fit with the wellness center's services, and what the level of effort involved will be if funds are received.

Depending upon the types of services provided, multiple small grants may be more helpful than one large grant. To manage a number of grants, the director should create a calendar with start and end dates, report due dates, and application due dates to assist the tracking process.

Contracts and Sub-Contracts

Some wellness centers have been quite successful at obtaining contracts from other community organizations and third-party payers to provide screening, health education, and referral services for specific populations. For example, one regional third-party payer hired the HPC to conduct blood pressure and cholesterol screenings at which there were counselors available to discuss Medicare Part D options. Some of these contracts are time-limited, and so are not the best source of continuing funding for a wellness center.

Sub-contracts can be very advantageous for a wellness center. A sub-contract is usually part of another agency's grant application. The other agency, in submitting a grant application in response to an RFP, requests funds to pay for sub-contracted services. The wellness center agrees to provide those services, then completes the grant sections related to the agreed upon scope of work. If the grant is approved and funded, the other agency issues a formal sub-contract for the work and pays from the grant funding. Tracking and reporting is done only for the services provided as outlined in the sub-contract, which is usually minimal compared to typical grant reporting. Because the HPC uses a partnership model, several community partners have included the HPC as a sub-contractor for specific services.

Donations

Donations can come from a variety of sources. Most important for wellness centers are corporate donations of funds and/or equipment, personal donations through combined giving (United Way, for example), and personal giving from people in the community.

Corporate donations represent an excellent source for equipment and other materials. Donations may come from small, local companies such as pharmacies and medical supply houses, or from larger corporations with which the partner university may have a connection. Every university has someone designated for corporate development who may provide information about companies in the region that may be willing to donate items that the wellness center might need.

The wellness center should consider placing information in the university alumni newsletter about the wellness center and combined giving. Most combined giving campaigns are required to allow the giver to designate where the donated funds must go. Ask alumni to designate your wellness center as the recipient, but make sure that the funds get placed into a specific account so donations can be tracked and the givers can be thanked. Some companies match individual donations, which multiplies each donation!

If the university is hesitant to designate the wellness center for combined giving, ask for a specific request of funds at another time of the year. Administration may need to be reminded that the wellness center is part of the university so, if they will not allow a specific request, ask how much the wellness center will receive from the annual university request.

People served in the community will often give something for the services they receive. Even if the services are offered for free, be sure to place a can for donations in a visible place. Any donations received must be placed in an active account for the wellness center and tracked through accounting within the university. Otherwise, it opens the center director to accusations of misuse of funds.

Sustainability

Sustainability rests on adequate and realistic planning. How much money is really needed to keep the wellness center open from year-to-year? Begin by building a bare bones budget. Given the goals of the wellness center and a realistic plan of operation, determine the least amount of funding needed to remain viable. This approach allows for a realistic appraisal of school and community resources needed to meet programmatic and community expectations. From this rudimentary budget, various budget projections can be constructed to demonstrate potential for growth and additional program development. This basic budget approach also allows administrators to recognize fall-back positions, should there be a gap in funding. It demonstrates that, even without substantial funding, the wellness center might be sustained.

Several factors contribute to the viability of a wellness center. These include space, services; recurring staff, equipment, site, and material costs; partners; and faculty and administrative support. Negotiate as long a contract for space as administration and the owner will allow. For example, opt for a three-year contract rather than a year-to-year contract for space. Plan for ideal space, but ask why the amount of space is needed. Wellness centers can be successful with limited space. Students are the primary source of labor through clinical service learning. Faculty may be sufficient to operate a wellness center on a part-time basis. Donated materials and equipment may be sufficient for start-up. And partners may be helpful in getting things started.

Faculty and administrative support are key to wellness center success. Each of these sectors must understand the goals of the wellness center as differentiated from those of a primary care center. The more faculty can integrate the goals of the center into specific courses, the greater the viability of the wellness center. Sustainability comes from institutionalizing the wellness center so that it becomes difficult to operate the school of nursing without it. It comes from having community partners who cannot fathom a community without wellness center services. And it comes from sustained funding from reliable sources, although those sources may change over time. Do not assume that initial support for the idea of a wellness center translates into sustainability. Work within the School or department to reach sustainability within the curriculum.

Most important in this process is that the leadership of the wellness center is committed to the university and school. Too often the wellness center is the work of one faculty member, so that the viability of the wellness center rests on that person's continuing involvement. Sustainability includes planning for succession—for someone who is the backup for the director and who can become the champion for the wellness center in the future.

Planning and Development of Independent Centers

Donna Torrisi, MSN

Tine Hansen-Turton, MGA, JD

Ann Deinhardt, MSW

8

A number of the contributors to this book represent larger organizations that, in addition to traditional wellness services, provide primary and mental/behavioral health care services. While many wellness centers work under the auspices of a school of nursing or a university, many of those that provide additional services are independent. During the initial stages of planning for a nurse-managed wellness center, it should be determined what services the center will provide and whether it will operate under a university, a hospital, or another non-profit organization, or whether it will be an independent non-profit 501(c)3, or even a for-profit corporation. This article will focus on the requirements if the center will offer primary or behavioral health services in addition to preventive and health promotion services, or if it will be a free-standing organization. Much of this information is derived from NNCC's book, *Community and Nurse-Managed Health Centers: Getting Them Started and Keeping Them Going,* written by Donna Torrisi and Tine Hansen-Turton and published by Springer in 2005. There is a startup checklist adapted to wellness centers in Appendix D-8.

Corporate Status

If a wellness center is to operate as a separate 501(c)3 organization, there is a significant amount of legal work to be accomplished. Assistance may be obtained from the NNCC, which might connect the new center with an experienced wellness center nearby, or from the university or potential partners, such as area hospitals. Filing for non-profit 501(c)3 status should be initiated as early as possible. Information on the process can be found at the IRS website, http://www.irs.gov/charities/index.html.

Governing Board

If the wellness center will operate as an independent organization, the governing board should be comprised of people who are committed to the mission of the wellness center and willing to work with management in decision-making and problem solving around the development and administration of the center. Board membership should be such that it represents and is able to serve as a link to the community that the center serves and reflects the interests and needs of the population. The board should have a diversity of strengths and capabilities to maximize its effectiveness. The types of skills needed should be identified at the outset and key community figures should be identified who will be able to help both in the development process and in identifying potential board members.

The board of an independent organization is governed through by-laws, which can be developed using those of another organization as a model and should be reviewed regularly. The roles to be taken by the governing board and the leadership need to be decided and spelled out in the by-laws. Minutes of board and committee meetings should be kept, even during initial planning meetings, distributed to all members and maintained, organized, and kept as a permanent and up-to-date record, including dates of meetings, names of participants, issues covered, and actions taken. As the organization matures, members of the board should receive formal orientation to the board and to the fiduciary and other responsibilities of membership, as well as to the center's mission, history, structure, goals, objectives, methods of operation, and key staff. New members should be provided with a Board Manual and encouraged to become familiar with the center.

Board Responsibilities—Mission, Executive Leadership, Oversight

The Board should conduct a thorough assessment of the area to be served in order to determine the resources available and the needs of the community. This process is addressed in the previous articles. The Board is responsible to develop the mission of the new organization. The mission should state whether the primary goal is to serve the community and/or to serve as a faculty practice or learning site for students, and whether the center will provide primary health services or health promotion services only. The mission and accompanying vision, principles, and/or values will help guide decision-making. The mission statement should be short and clear and should convey the vision of the center to clients, staff, funders, and the community. The services to be provided will flow from the mission and the needs of the community that are determined through the needs assessment.

A governing board is responsible for the selection, evaluation, and, where necessary, dismissal of the CEO or Director to whom it delegates authority and responsibility for the organization's management. The Board is also responsible for the fiduciary oversight of the organization, including assuring that adequate insurance is carried, that sound fiscal practices are being followed, and that fiscal audits and program monitoring are being carried out. To this end, the Board approves policies that guide the work of the organization and promote sound business practices, consistency of performance, and communication of standards and expectations to the staff. There should also be a quality improvement program in place to assure that services are high quality and meeting clients' needs. These are discussed in one of the previous articles. It is the responsibility of the Director to assist in the development of these policies and to see that they are carried out. The Board should receive reports from the Executive Director regarding the operation and finances of the center and progress made toward strategic plan goals a minimum of four times a year. The boardsource website is an excellent source of information about boards, including resources that can be tailored to the needs of each center (http://www.boardsource.org/).

Site Selection, Zoning, and Licensing

Once the mission and services to be provided are determined, a site must be selected. The site needs to be accessible to the target population, available by public transportation in most instances, and adequate for the services to be provided. The center may be free-standing or located in a partner organization's facility. The facility or building may need to be zoned for the type of services to be provided. Zoning is the way government controls the physical development of land and uses of property. Even though a space may have commercial zoning, it is important to know whether or not it can be utilized as a health-related facility. As mentioned earlier, it is advisable to contact state and local political entities, as well as a lawyer, early in the process to assure that sites being considered are viable possibilities.

It is important for the organization to obtain any licenses required for the services and the facility. Requirements vary from state by state. The Center Director will need to contact the state's health department for requirements. A list of the State Boards of Nursing, where information may also be available, can be found at www.allnursingschools.com/faqs/boards.php. In addition to licensing the services and the facility, the director of the center must verify that employees are certified or licensed as necessary. Copies of the nurse-practitioners' current certifications and/or state licenses should be on file, as should any practice agreement with a collaborating physician that may be required, depending on the services to be provided. If mental health services are to be provided, the appropriate licenses for this service and the providers must be maintained.

Funding

The financial development process requires a great deal of flexibility and creativity. Finding nontraditional sources of funding, such as private philanthropic foundations and corporations is important because the pillars of public health: health promotion, health education, and disease prevention, are often not reimbursed by public sources or patients. Also, it is important for nurse-managed health and wellness centers to cultivate multiple funding streams, to the degree possible, in order to have adequate cash flow and to be viable.

Obtaining a major grant can secure the finances of a center for the length of the grant. Such funding can enhance the center's public image and may leverage other funding as well. Grants from local public entities, such as health departments, may provide reliable and predictable income for the wellness center. Before seeking grant funding, the center should complete its strategic plan, as many funders require such a plan before considering a grant, particularly for a new organization or new program. Descriptions (sometimes called case statements) should be developed regarding the specific programs or items for which funding will be requested, including a full discussion of the need for the services, details of services to be provided, outcomes to be achieved, and methods of evaluation to be used.

Many wellness centers provide services for which patients and/or third party payers can be charged fees. In setting fees, health centers must find a balance between fees that are adequate to cover the cost of services and the need to avoid over-pricing of services. The fee-for-service model requires a billing and collection system and the development of a sliding scale fee schedule for patients who are uninsured or underinsured.

Contracts with public entities or other organizations, such as service agencies, businesses, unions, or housing authorities, may provide reliable and predictable income for the health and wellness center as payment for specific services. Public contracts usually come with a great deal of oversight and regulation. Contracts with both public and private organizations must be constructed carefully to assure that they are specific about services that are covered and those that may be separate from the contract. Contracts should detail the ways in which services are paid for and cover the ways that disputes are negotiated. Contracts are binding and must be adhered to even if resources or staffing declines, unless both parties renegotiate the terms. See Appendix D-8 for a sample of a contract with a local agency.

Conclusion

In order for the nurse-managed health and wellness center model to continue to flourish, technical support is needed for the development of new centers and the growth of the existing ones. The NNCC Guide, *Community and Nurse-Managed Health Centers: Getting Them Started and Keeping Them Going*, can be helpful as a resource for people or organizations that are interested in starting new independent centers or growing those that are currently providing solely wellness services. It can help a center to address issues of sustainability and questions such as whether to seek accreditation or Federally Qualified Health Center (FQHC) status.

Resources

http://www.boardsource.org

www.allnursingschools.com/faqs/boards.php

Torrisi, D. L., & Hansen-Turton, T. (2005). *Community and Nurse-Managed Health Centers: Getting Them Started and Keeping Them Going*. New York: Springer Publishing Company.

Wellness
Center
Services

Traditional Wellness Center Services

Ann C. Deinhardt, MSW

Tine Hansen-Turton, MGA, JD

Nancy Rothman, EdD, RN

Sormeh Harounzadeh

Nurse-managed wellness centers provide a tremendous diversity of services in a variety of settings. Some centers are "center-based," working in a free-standing facility or in space within another service organization. Others are centers "without walls," which provide services throughout their communities. Services include providing extensive outreach and working in schools, housing developments, people's homes, and other community venues. Although all wellness centers provide disease screenings and health education, centers often focus on specific populations, across the life cycles, specific jobs or workplaces, and a variety of specific problems. In addition to providing services, they are often active in their communities, doing outreach at community events and advocating for appropriate supports for children, youth, seniors, and families, including education, economic security, work opportunities, transportation, housing, and other necessary services, in recognition that these supports greatly impact people's health. Their partnerships with local agencies and government bodies are very important to wellness centers, as is clear in the profiles found in Appendices A and B.

Wellness centers offer care to a broad spectrum of patients and tackle common health issues, using education and screening to decrease the experience of preventable health complications in the community and to help people manage their chronic illnesses. One person indicated that wellness centers provide every kind of health service imaginable other than primary care. However, a number of the centers featured in this book do provide primary and mental/behavioral health services, but these centers continue to focus on health promotion and disease prevention services and consider themselves to be both wellness and primary health care centers.

Wellness centers services can be grouped into four categories:

- Health teaching, guidance, and counseling, e.g., diabetes education, cardiovascular health, dental care education, safety education, and health and life management;
- Surveillance, e.g., height and weight measurement, vision and hearing screening, glucose monitoring, and blood pressure evaluation;
- Immunizations; and
- Administration of treatments and procedures, e.g., wound care and first aid.

Wellness centers serve people across the life cycles, providing a variety of health services. The NNCC, as well as its members, have developed a number of health promotion programs based on best practices, which are discussed at the end of this chapter.

Wellness Center Services for the Life Cycles

Maternal Health

Education is an extremely important component of maternal health care. Pregnant women need information about what to expect during and after their pregnancy. Wellness centers work in communities, often in partnership with prenatal care clinics or public housing, where many women of childbearing age are likely to be found, to educate women who are pregnant or may become pregnant. Education topics may include diet, exercise, the birth process, breast-feeding, and newborn care. Women might also be offered information about post-partum depression, domestic violence, prevention of sexually transmitted infections, and family planning. Some centers participate in the national Nurse-Family Partnership program, providing home visiting by a public health nurse and intensive case management to women and families during their first pregnancy and through the second year of the baby's life. Others provide promontora de salud paraprofessional services to help new mothers. These services are offered with the goal of supporting women's prenatal care and improving health outcomes for them and their infants.

Infant and Child Health

Just as with pregnant women, wellness centers work to assure that mothers, infants, and children receive the medical care they need and help to connect them with providers. Screenings that might be conducted include height and weight, vision, and hearing, as well as screening for dental problems. Other infant and child services may include health education for child care programs, immunizations, fitness education and programming such as summer camps that have a health focus and literacy promotion programs, such as Reach Out and Read that provides a new book for children at well-child visits and educates parents about the value of reading to children. Information or referrals may be made to such community services as domestic violence shelter and counseling, behavioral health and drug and alcohol treatment programs, parenting training, WIC and food assistance, income assistance resources, education services and work-related programs, housing-related and legal resources, and cultural, enrichment, and recreation services.

Some wellness centers that are focused on infants and children conduct screenings for signs of lead poisoning, autism, and other problems or delays in child development that might require early intervention. Screening for lead poisoning can alert families to home hazards and families can be helped to prevent any further exposure to a lead-hazardous environment. Information about a safe home environment can be provided, including information on lead poisoning and how to prevent it. Some centers use the NNCC program, Lead Safe Babies, which is designed to teach new mothers about lead poisoning and test their homes for lead dust that could potentially be harmful. The program provides some home repairs on an as-needed basis and is offered to all new mothers in the Philadelphia area. A similar program is Asthma Safe Kids, in which home visits are made by outreach workers to educate children and parents about asthma prevention and care.

Developmental screening tools used in some nurse-managed health centers include the M-CHAT, which screens for autism and can be found at www.firstsigns.org. This tool is for toddlers between 16 and 30 months of age, and is used to assess risk for autism spectrum disorders (ASD). Children who fail more than three items should be referred for early intervention. Centers can use behavioral development screening tools such as the Denver Developmental Test and the Ages and Stages Questionnaire. These tests assess children's fine motor, gross motor, language, and cognitive skills and can be used with infants to children up to six years of age. Information on the Denver Test can be found at www.denverii.com. The Ages and Stages Questionnaires are done in partnership with the parents, offering them information about what to expect from their children at various developmental stages. Information on this system can be found at www.agesandstages.com. Again, wellness centers facilitate families' connection to medical, early intervention, or social services as needed. Some provide services to children with health problems and special needs, and their at-risk families, including family and environmental home assessment, educational visits, and referrals to community agencies.

Youth Health

Nutrition and exercise are significant education points for children and adolescents. Parents may be offered classes in fitness and nutrition and meal planning and preparation, as well as joint programs with their children in these areas, such as HRSA's BodyWorks, an evidence-based program that promotes healthy eating and physical activity for girls, ages 9 to 13 years, and their mothers.

A number of centers use NNCC's Students Run Philly Style, a long-distance running and mentoring program for youth. The program holds races throughout the year for students and matches students with adult mentors who help them reach their goals and perform well in school.

Health and wellness centers may have space and be able to provide a number of programs to help young people in the community make choices that will result in better health. Some of these might include G.I.R.L.S. (Gaining Independence Rebuilding Lives Successfully), which addresses issues on "growing up female" including date rape and self-esteem; Peaceful Posse, which works with boys around issues of violence; and other skills and health programs that provide screening and counseling services for adolescents around sexual health, safety, school performance, work life, and depression and behavioral health.

Adult Health

Wellness care for adults is a broad area of practice. A wellness center can provide screenings for heart disease, stroke, diabetes, breast cancer, prostate cancer, and cervical cancer, as well as education about these conditions and how to prevent and detect them. Tobacco cessation and exercise promotion programs, such as the NNCCs Tobacco Cessation and Stay Quit Get Fit, and others such as the *salsaerobics* exercise classes discussed in one of the articles below, can offer adults resources and guidance to make healthy decisions. NNCCs programs provide free nicotine replacement therapy, information brochures, and counseling services. The *salsaerobics* are combined with health assessments, referrals for services, and an integrated chronic disease prevention curriculum. The latter is successful because it specifically addresses the culture of the people served, a factor that must be taken into consideration when developing any wellness services.

Wellness centers can provide support groups to promote healthy outcomes for people with chronic conditions. People with diabetes can benefit from support groups where they can learn about managing their illness and overcoming the barriers to health that they face. People living with cancer and their families can support each other as well. Other groups can serve people with depression and people in recovery. Some centers partner with or provide space for groups such as AA and NA. Some centers also collaborate with homeless shelters or services for people with mental illness to provide health screenings and education to people using these services.

Senior Health

Many wellness centers work with senior centers, senior housing, and other organizations that work with older people living in the community. Some provide home visits and conduct home safety and functioning assessments; screenings for depression, tobacco use and use of drug and alcohol; and referrals to medical specialty care, dental, legal, housing and other services, as needed. Other centers conduct screening for high blood pressure, diabetes, and obesity; nutrition and cooking classes; immunization clinics; medication brown bag days, where people can bring in their medications and receive assistance in understanding their regimen and any drug interactions to avoid; and services to help older people manage their health and prescription insurance coverage. Some of these services have been found to contribute directly to enabling older adults to manage their health issues and sustain functional independence. Other services get people out of their homes, into social situations, and involved in the community. Fitness programs, lecture series, and computer classes all provide seniors with access to information, including health information, that can greatly enrich their lives.

Best Practices: Promoting Healthy Living and Meeting People's Health Needs

Approximately 65% of the funding NNCC raises through grants goes directly to member health centers. Over the past eight years, NNCC has successfully developed several signature health promotion programs that it contracts with member centers to provide. NNCC also administers the national Nurse-Family Partnership for several member agencies in Philadelphia. The Temple Health Connection has also developed several innovative programs that are discussed below.

The Nurse-Family Partnership provides client-centered home visiting services by nurses to first-time, low-income eligible mothers. The services are designed to ensure that mothers will have healthier pregnancies, child health and development will be improved, and mothers will become more self-sufficient. Recognized by the RAND Corporation as an evidence-based program, the Nurse-Family Partnership has more than 30 years of data to support its powerful results. Philadelphia's program is part of the national network of Nurse-Family Partnerships, which all apply the evaluated model. Since 2001, the Nurse-Family Partnership has served over 1600 women in Philadelphia (400 women each 30-month program cycle).

The NNCC Cognitive Therapy Program is a partnership with the Beck Institute for Cognitive Therapy and Research, which promotes the incorporation of cognitive behavioral therapy (CBT) into health care and counseling in a range of settings, including primary care offices, schools, and community-based service organizations. The NNCC has provided training for nurses on how to incorporate CBT into their health care regimens. CBT is a psychotherapy approach that prompts changes in thinking, actions, and emotional responses by problem solving in the present. Over 375 outcome studies have shown CBT to be highly effective for treating many mental health problems, including depression, general anxiety disorder, and substance abuse. In 2005, nurses involved in the program had a 27% improvement on a test of cognitive therapy awareness and elderly patients had a 28% decrease in anxiety scores.

NNCC's Asthma Safe Kids Program helps improve the living conditions of asthmatic children by eliminating asthma triggers in the children's home environment through education and in-home assessment. As a result, children have fewer asthma attacks and fewer emergency room visits and hospitalizations. Education and assessment materials are based upon the American Lung Association's *Attack Asthma* curriculum, and the Environmental Protection Agency's Home Environmental Assessment. These have been adapted to teach parents about how to address asthma triggers in their own home. Caregivers also receive trigger-reduction supplies, such as mattress covers and roach bait. In 2007, children in the program had an 8% reduction in emergency room visits in the past six months and a 14% reduction in smoking within their homes.

The NNCC has a number of Lead Poisoning Prevention programs that approach this problem from many angles: reaching out to low-income, new or expecting mothers through presentations at service agencies (e.g., WIC offices); contacting all new families in Philadelphia through new birth data; and referring pregnant mothers or families with infants into NNCC's evidence-based prevention program, Lead Safe Babies.

- Lead Safe Babies educates new mothers and fathers on how to avoid lead poisoning for their children. Since the year 2000, over 7,000 Philadelphia families have received education on how to prevent lead poisoning, including an in-home assessment for the presence of lead. In 2005, the Environmental Protection Agency recognized Lead Safe Babies with its Children's Environmental Health award. In 2007, there was a 42% relative risk reduction in blood lead levels for children in the program compared to children living within the same census tract block groups.
- The Lead Safe Homes Study examines different ways to prevent lead poisoning in newborns and young children. The study educates parents of participating children on lead exposure and how to keep a child safe from lead poisoning, testing the amount and type of intervention needed to keep children lead free.
- LeadSafe DC provides families in Washington, DC with education about lead poisoning prevention for their children, successfully replicating the Lead Safe Babies program in our nation's capitol. The Director of Lead-Safe DC facilitates an inter-agency Lead Elimination Task Force, which brings together federal, regional, and local stakeholders to create strategies, form partnerships and leverage resources to attack the problem of lead poisoning.

NNCC's newest program, First Steps for Autism, helps families connect with local community resources and have access to up-to-date information pertaining to Autism and available services. First Steps staff make home visits to low-income families with a child suspected of having or diagnosed with an Autism Spectrum Disorder. Staff help the family develop a plan, and then coordinate visits from a variety of clinicians. First Steps also trains providers and child caregivers regarding appropriate developmental assessment.

Healthy Homes for Childcare provides assessment, education, and physical remediation to licensed home-based childcare providers to help them ensure a healthy and safe environment for children. Healthy Homes for Childcare is a collaboration between the Pennsylvania Department of Public Welfare, the Philadelphia Department of Public Health, the NNCC, and other nonprofit agencies in Philadelphia.

Heart & Soul is an interactive NNCC health education program focused on heart-healthy living. Heart & Soul is a nutrition and exercise program encouraging women, men, and youth to adopt healthy lifestyle changes, including disease management, good eating habits, and regular exercise. Classes are held in a variety of community venues, such as residential treatment centers and after school programs.

The NNCC Students Run Philly Style is the only program in Philadelphia that offers marathon training to help young people succeed in life. Students Run Philly Style connects students with adult mentors who help them imagine and accomplish goals beyond their dreams, including the completion of a marathon. The program helps youth go farther: encouraging youth to be healthy for life, to make safe choices, and to do well in school. In 2008, participants had a statistically significant reduction in body mass index.

NNCC sponsors two Tobacco Cessation efforts:

- Stay Quit, Get Fit integrates smoking cessation counseling, primary care, and exercise classes for low-income African American adults at a nurse-managed health center in North Philadelphia. Primary care providers reinforce cessation messages and address chronic health conditions exacerbated by tobacco use.
- Be Free From Nicotine is a six-week program that helps smokers get ready to quit, quit smoking, and learn how to stay tobacco free. The program, run by a certified counselor, provides free nicotine patches, gum, and lozenges, as well as stress reduction and relaxation skills to participants.

The Southwest Breast Health Initiative helps people to understand that early screening and detection are essential in combating breast cancer. Research has established that women in minority populations are less likely to receive screening, detect breast cancer early, and hence have higher mortality rates. This NNCC initiative provides incentives and access to women in the neighborhoods of southwest Philadelphia that are primarily African-American to receive clinical breast exams and mammograms.

Women Go Red Philly Style works to improve the heart health of African-American women in places where Philadelphia women work, live, and receive their health care. This NNCC program trains health care providers working in low-income communities regarding current clinical guidelines for cardiovascular risk assessment and treatment of women. It also educates women in community, health care, and workplace settings about how to reduce their risk of cardiovascular disease. Women Go Red Philly Style encourages integrating policies that promote cardiovascular health into key aspects of daily life.

In the Temple Health Connection March of Dimes Breastfeeding Support Center, outreach workers hired from the community facilitated support groups and visited expectant mothers and new mothers in clinics, the hospital, and their homes. Tee-shirts which read, "I'm Happier, I'm Smarter, I'm Healthier Because My Mother Breastfed Me!" were given to new moms who breastfeed for three months. At an annual Breastfeeding Celebration, held during International Breastfeeding Week, LaRhona Upshur, a Philadelphia radio personality, was the MC and her station, Power 99, broadcasted from the event to let listeners know the benefits of breastfeeding.

For the Anti Tobacco Outreach Program, Temple Health Connection joined forces with the Center for Intergenerational Learning's Full Circle Theater to apply for anti-tobacco funds. Student nurses worked with inner-city high school students to research and publicize the media ploys of large tobacco companies and the dangers of second-hand smoke. Large murals and poster contests for all city children were the direct result of brainstorming by the students and the community advisory board. The City secured money to shrink-wrap buses with the winning posters.

Conclusion

The articles that follow cover services focused specifically on older people and Latinos, and behavioral health services. Together and with the organizational profiles found in the appendices, these can give schools or organizations that are thinking of opening a wellness center a wealth of ideas for services that can be provided.

Resources

www.agesandstages.com
www.denverii.com
www.firstsigns.org
www.nncc.us/programs

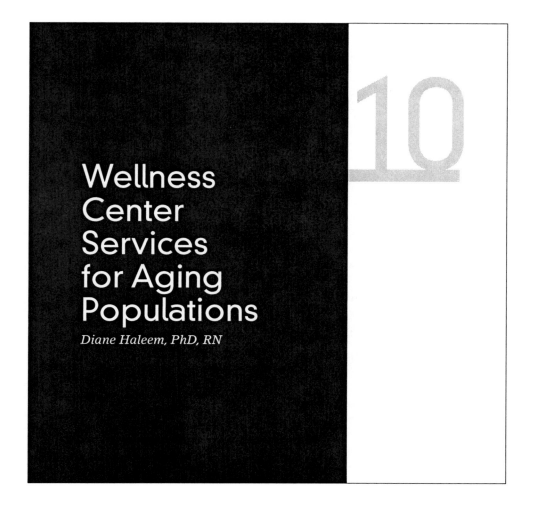

Wellness Center Services for Aging Populations

Diane Haleem, PhD, RN

Aging Stats 1900s–2020

In the early 1900s, there were 3.1 million elderly in the United States. About one in twenty-five Americans was elderly. The elderly population in 2020 is projected to increase to 54 million persons, and about one in six Americans would be elderly. More children would know their great grandparents, as the four-generation family would become more common. There were 122,000 persons 85 years old and over in 1900, less than one percent of the population, and the average life expectancy for persons born in 1900 was 47 years. It is projected in 2020, about 6.5 million persons will be 85 years old and over (U.S. Department of Commerce, Economics and Statistics Administration, Bureau of the Census, 1993). Impressive numbers!

With an increased number of people living longer, there are a greater number of health problems that need to be managed. The following programs are designed to help people keep their minds and bodies at optimal health. Health promotion activities at and coordinated by Wellness Centers can be an invaluable service to the elder population. The following provides ideas as well as resources to conduct meaningful activities with people of age to address their health and well-being.

Activities Addressing Health and Well-Being of the Elderly

Day Activities at a wellness center can offer people of age opportunities to engage with other people, socializing and interacting with other members of the community. Participants can engage in programs such as book clubs, mental fitness activities, nutrition awareness, spiritual wellness programs, and exercise.

Nutrition Awareness

Eating healthy is important to physical and mental health. The Food and Nutrition Information Center has a wonderful Web site with excellent resources and provides tips for eating healthfully (National Agricultural Library, 2007). This 36-page document gives a wealth of information and resources. It covers three sections. 1) General Health and Nutrition, 2) Resources by format—books, cookbooks and recipes, and newsletters, as well as nutrition and health organizations by topic, for example, arthritis, cancer, diabetes, and osteoporosis. The American Academy of Family Physicians provides a screening tool, "Determine Your Nutritional Health," that can be used to assess a person's nutritional health (see Appendix D-11). Assisting people of age in completing this tool can be a first step in having someone determine if they are at risk. Knowing their risk factors is useful in developing an action plan to address their needs.

Eating Well as We Age

Many older adults have difficulty maintaining good nutrition as a result of decreased appetite, difficulty chewing, and other problems. Having educational sessions that give practical tips to address the possible challenges of eating well can help facilitate solutions to practical problems. The U.S. Department of Health and Human Services Food and Drug Administration Web site provides resources on how to address and overcome six nutritional concerns, including 1) can't chew, 2) upset stomach, 3) shopping, 4) cooking, 5) no appetite, and 6) short on money (U.S. Department of Health and Human Services, Food and Drug Administration, 2006).

Some of the practical solutions suggested include:

Problem: Can't Shop

- Ask the local food store to bring groceries to your home. Some stores deliver free. Sometimes there is a charge.
- Ask your church or synagogue for volunteer help or sign up for help with a local volunteer center.
- Ask a family member or neighbor to shop for you or pay someone to do it. Some companies let you hire home health workers for a few hours a week. These workers may shop for you, and do other things. Look for these companies in the Yellow Pages of the phone book under "Home Health Services."

Problem: Can't Cook

- Use a microwave oven to cook TV dinners, other frozen foods, and prepared foods from the grocery store.
- Take part in group meal programs, offered through senior citizen programs or have meals brought to your home.

▓ Move to a place where someone else will cook, such as a family member's home or a home for senior citizens.

Problem: No Appetite

▓ Eat with family and friends.
▓ Take part in group meal programs, offered through senior citizen programs.
▓ Ask your doctor if your medicines could be causing appetite or taste problems. If so, ask about changing medicines.
▓ Increase the flavor of food by adding spices and herbs.

Problem: Short on Money

▓ Buy low-cost food, such as dried beans, peas, rice, and pasta, or buy food that contains these items, such as split pea soup, canned beans, and rice.
▓ Use coupons for discounts on foods you like.
▓ Buy foods on sale. Also buy store-brand foods, as they often cost less.
▓ Find out if your local church or synagogue offers free or low-cost meals.
▓ Take part in group meal programs, offered through local senior citizen programs. Or have these meals brought to your home.
▓ Get food stamps. Call the food stamp office listed under your county government in the blue pages of the phone book.

Cooking-Healthy Classes

Weekly cooking classes can take place with demonstrations and tastings. Recipes can be shared with participants to take home and try. Each week can focus on a different topic that addresses healthy eating. Participants can bring in recipes and samples of their favorite healthy dishes to share with fellow participants. This is often a very popular heavily attended program.

Exercise: Fit and Fabulous as You Mature

In 2005–2006, 22% of people age 65 and over reported engaging in regular physical activity. The percentage of older people engaging in regular physical activity was lower at older ages, ranging from 26% among people age 65–74, and 10% among people age 85 and over (AgingStats.gov, 2008).

Staying fit is important. Information people need to know includes the fact that being overweight can lead to a greater risk of developing:

▓ diabetes
▓ coronary heart disease
▓ high blood cholesterol
▓ stroke
▓ hypertension
▓ gallbladder disease
▓ osteoarthritis (degeneration of cartilage and bone of joints)
▓ sleep apnea and other breathing problems
▓ some forms of cancer (breast, colorectal, endometrial, and kidney)

(U. S. Department of Health and Human Services, National Institute of Health, 2007).

Fit and Fabulous classes stress that exercise is not only healthful for physical health but also mental health. Exercise can help reduce stress, help you feel better about yourself, give you energy, and relieve boredom. Developing an exercise program specifically for your age is essential. Exercise can be both fun and engaging. Dancing is a great source of exercise. There are programs and resources that can help get you started and stay motivated. They can also improve and maintain your endurance, strength, balance, and flexibility. Questions like, "What can exercise do for me? Is it safe for me to exercise? How to keep going?" are important questions that can be answered in, "Exercise: a Guide from The National Institute on Aging" (2004, Reprinted April, 2008). The U.S. Department of Health and Human Services and the National Institute of Health are agencies that provide resources and tips for exercise plans and offer helpful information on nutrition and meal preparation.

Mental Fitness

The focus of mental fitness programs is to keep people of age engaged. Mental fitness can be accomplished in many ways. A great way to practice mental fitness is through a book club where participants have periodic meetings to discuss books and their contents. Books can include healthy living choices such as:

- Essential Concepts for Healthy Living by Sandra Alters;
- Living a Healthy Life with Chronic Conditions: Self-Management of Heart Disease, Fatigue, Arthritis, Worry, Diabetes, Frustration, Asthma, Pain, Emphysema, and others by Kate Lorig, Halsted Holman, David Sobel, and Diana Laurent, and Nutrition for Health Living by Wendy Schiff.

For those who can't read or are challenged by reading, a volunteer program can be organized to read out loud to participants. Board games such as Scrabble, Jeopardy, and Wheel of Fortune can be used to stimulate the mind. Activities where students engage in conversation with people of age is also a wonderful experience both for the students and the elderly participants. Stimulating the mind is an invaluable activity.

Keeping Informed

There are many online resources that provide access to health-related topics. Wellness centers can provide computer classes, possibly in coordination with the local library. The information available on the Internet is tremendous. Giving people access to this information provides them a wealth of knowledge on health and wellness.

Other Health Promotion Activities

The possibilities for educational activities that are fun and informative are endless. Some ideas and subjects could include learning to recognize early signs of illness; substance use, alcohol, and prescribed medications; emotional wellness, using music; spiritual wellness; and stress awareness and management.

Cultivate a wellness library consisting of educational videos, pamphlets, and CDs that can be checked out.

Blood Pressure Screenings: What Every Older Adult Should Know
People over 55 have a 90% chance of developing high blood pressure. The National Heart Lung and Blood Institute's Web site provides information about high blood pressure and tips for preventing heart disease, including eight things older people can do to prevent and control high blood pressure. The eight prevention tips are: 1) Lose weight, 2) Eat heart-healthy, 3) Reduce salt and sodium intake, 4) Drink any alcoholic beverage in moderation, 5) Become more physically fit, 6) Quit smoking, 7) Talk with your health care professional, and 8) Take your medicine as prescribed (The National High Blood Pressure Education Program, 2004). Having screenings and education programs addressing blood pressure can be a tremendous help in addressing and controlling blood pressure.

Flu Shots
The Centers for Disease Control recommends that people 50 years of age and older and people of any age with certain chronic medical conditions (such as asthma, diabetes, or heart disease), as well as people who live in nursing homes and other long-term care facilities, have annual flu shots. Influenza (commonly known as the flu) is easily transmitted from person to person. Unlike the common cold, it can leave a person unable to function for several days, particularly an older person. Getting an annual vaccination is the best protection from the flu and its debilitating effects (The Centers for Disease Control, 2008). Having a flu clinic can be a great way to maintain the health of a person with age. Some facilities do a drive-by clinic, where the person does not need to step out of their car. The health professional can come to the car, complete the appropriate paperwork, and give the person their injection while still in the car.

Medication Teaching
Have a day where each person of age brings in all of his or her medications. Ask the patients if they know what the medications are for, what the side effects are, and when they need to take the medications. This is an excellent way to do medication teaching. If there are any questions from the health care professional running this session, these can be written down for the participants to follow up with their health provider.

Outreach to people living in their homes or facilities can also be done. For those who are unable to leave their residence or find it difficult, home visits to review their medications can be invaluable. This also gives the health care professional an opportunity to suggest any aids or other assistive programs that the person would benefit from (i.e., Meals on Wheels, home health visits, etc.).

Help!

Don't hesitate to contact schools and solicit nursing students to help with some programs. Intergenerational engagement is very positive. Also seek out retired nurses who want to volunteer their time and experience.

Resources

Older Adults

http://www.nal.usda.gov/fnic/pubs/olderadults.pdf - addressing nutrition, health organizations, diabetes, and osteoporosis.

Eating Well

http://www.fda.gov/opacom/lowlit/eatage.html

Exercise

http://win.niddk.nih.gov/publications/mature.htm

http://win.niddk.nih.gov/publications/PDFs/FitandFabulous2004.pdf

http://www.niapublications.org/exercisebook/ExerciseGuideComplete.pdf

http://win.niddk.nih.gov/statistics/index.htm

http://www.niapublications.org/exercisebook/ExerciseGuideComplete.pdf

Blood Pressure

http://hp2010.nhlbihin.net/mission/partner/midlife.pdf

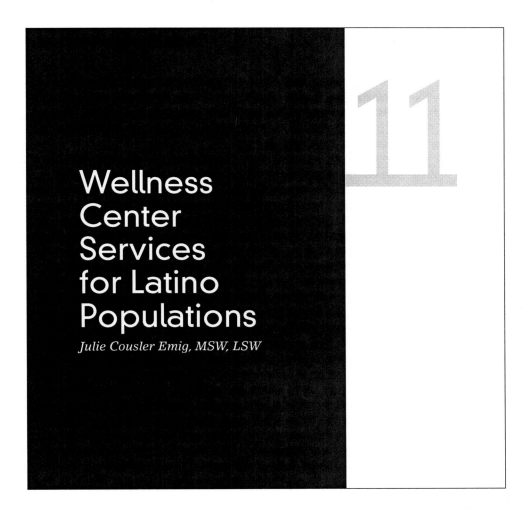

11

Wellness Center Services for Latino Populations

Julie Cousler Emig, MSW, LSW

Overview of Services to Latinos

According to the United States Census Bureau's 2006 American Community Survey, Latinos, or Hispanics, account for nearly 15% of the country's population, a 26% increase since 2000 (2006). Latinos represent an ethnically and culturally diverse group comprised of foreign born (40%) and native born (60%) residents (Pew Hispanic Center, 2006). Latinos enrich our society in many ways, growing our palate with good foods, our sense of collectivism with a strong commitment to family, and our appreciation for life and others through cultural emphasis on respect (*respeto*), personal relationships (*personalismo*), and trust or friendliness (*confianza*). Yet Latinos also challenge our national sense of public health and well-being with poor health outcomes surpassing most other groups, particularly within certain sub-groups by country of origin. This chapter explores the key components of effective health promotion strategies targeting Latinos, and one Latino community-based organization's success with program models that address a variety of pressing public health concerns.

Many Latino populations are insulated geographically and socially, where most of their needs are met within the community and in their native tongue of

Spanish. This supports newcomers in the acclimation process and grows a valu-able sense of community, but it also challenges the professional and academic community's desire to bring promising and best practices to Latinos. Partner-ship with Latino community-based organizations, or patience and persistence in becoming a part of the community, is key.

Service providers to Latinos must earn the trust of the community. People will share their successful experience with a provider with their friends and family and a provider's prominence in the community will grow. For most pro-viders, this trust grows over time and patience is important. Services to Latinos need to be offered in their native language of Spanish to accommodate and welcome a community with broad and varying levels of English proficiency, although it should be noted that a variety of indigenous dialects may present from many countries like Mexico and Guatemala, complicating communication significantly. Latinos also need to feel comfortable in the space where services are offered, and the site needs to be close and easily accessible. Traditional artwork adorning walls and bright colors common to Latino countries and com-munities help to welcome and set the stage for comfort.

Establishing trust with the community requires cultural competency or proficiency among staff and in organizational practices. Language and embrac-ing cultural norms builds cultural competency. The cultural norms of *respeto,* *personalismo,* and *confianza,* and those of espiritú, the integrated health approach based on an understanding of a greater power (God) having a role in the approach of healing the body, mind, and spirit, and machismo and mari-anismo, traditional gender roles, should be embraced for the strong value that they have in the community and the power that they hold in influencing good health and social outcomes. Many Americans wrongly believe that machismo is a negative norm that equates to aggressiveness and dominance. While it does carry this negative connotation in some exaggerated and unhealthy circles, it more appropriately and globally means responsibility. Latino men are usually seen as the head of the household and have a strong sense of commitment to provide for and protect their family. Latino women tend to be the nurturers of the family, assuming the responsibilities of the home, including the extended family's health care, sometimes at the neglect of their own. All of these norms are healthy and powerful influencers of health and well-being and should be embraced by providers as strengths upon which to build.

An important way to build cultural competency in services is to employ staff that mirror the community. Bilingual and bicultural staff helps to build trust and help design programming and interventions that are congruent with Latino norms and values. They also serve as role models for community mem-bers. The need for professional competency of those staff is implicit, although that doesn't always mean formal post-secondary education. Formal education is often necessary among staff delivering interventions, depending on the degree of sophistication of the program or demand for analytical skills, but it isn't always necessary. Professional health program staffing can often be enhanced or augmented by promotoras, or health promoters, who intimately understand and are of the culture, and can communicate messages in ways that the com-munity can relate to and envision incorporation for themselves. Hiring promo-toras or non-professional staff, and professional staff for that matter, requires an assessment process during hiring to ensure that prospective staff shares the values, ethics, and consciousness necessary to influence the community toward desired outcomes. Ongoing staff development is also critical for lay and professional Latino staff where English is often their second language.

Lastly, the importance of input from the community as programming is developed cannot be overstated. No one knows better than the service consumers what will work in achieving desired impact. Focus groups and key informant interviews can help providers tailor interventions and activities to Latinos, learning what will work and won't work while building consciousness of the proposed service among participants. Each of the program models highlighted below was developed with some level of participant input. Each was developed with or by a Philadelphia-based Latino multi-service organization, Congreso de Latinos Unidos. Founded in 1977 by a group of Puerto Rican activists, Congreso today serves nearly 20,000 people annually with direct services across health, workforce development, youth, and family domains. Each model highlighted below was chosen for its innovative approach to Latino health promotion, and for its proven impact.

Promising Approaches

Chronic Disease Prevention & Early Intervention Programming

In 1997, Congreso founded its Women's Center, actualized by a group of committed clients from the domestic violence and maternal and child health programs, who sought to illuminate the path for other women struggling with challenges similar to theirs. Five years later, capitalizing on the power of the Center in attracting women facing like barriers, a captive audience, *Proyecto Salud* was founded. *Proyecto Salud* (Health Project) formalized the sewing and cooking classes, and the newer *salsaerobics* exercise classes with 16-week class modules that included established, comprehensive assessment and related service referrals, an integrated chronic disease prevention curriculum, and measurement of outcomes and desired impact. Ideally, women progressed through all three different classes across 48 weeks for sustained learning and impact, and the promotion of promotoras carried on health messages.

Focused on cardiovascular health, diabetes, obesity, mental health, and domestic violence, pressing health issues for Latinos from Congreso's community, the *Proyecto Salud* curriculum was developed using Spanish health education materials, largely from the National Alliance for Hispanic Health, the American Diabetes and Heart Associations, the National Institutes for Health and Mental Health, and ALIANZA, the National Latino Alliance for the Elimination of Domestic Violence. Between 15 and 40 women participated in each class (sewing, cooking, *Latino Meals Made Healthy*, and salsaerobics), with approximately 240 served in total annually.

Cardiac and metabolic risk factors related to cardiovascular disease and diabetes measured were body mass index (BMI) and blood pressure. Salsaerobics participants were further measured for change in waist-to-hip ratio and abdominal obesity. Psychosocial risk factors measured for all participants were depressive symptoms, using the Center for Epidemiological Studies depression scale (CES-D), and perceived social support, via self-report. Results in the salsaerobics exercise class indicated decreases in both BMI and abdominal obesity, and results across all three classes indicated decreases in symptoms of depression and increases in social support among Latinas who completed the program. Those who did not complete the program were younger, had greater depressive symptomatology, reported poorer social support, and they tended to be caregivers and U.S. born. More information on these data can be found in a paper published in the *Journal for Community Health,* titled "Un Corazon Saludable: Factors Influencing Outcomes of an Exercise Program Designed to Impact Cardiac and Metabolic Risks among Urban Latinas" (Harralson et al., 2007).

Focus groups were used annually to enhance the program. In year two, a grant was obtained from the local Kynett and Barra Foundations to integrate case management services, based on the overwhelming need for service connection and early intervention in a host of areas learned through the assessment and screening for depressive symptoms and health indicators. Women repeatedly said that they wanted to exercise with their children, so *Ninos Saludable* (Healthy Children) was developed in 2006, which was salsaerobics tailored to caregivers and children together. The associated educational curriculum was based on Washington State's Healthy Choices for Kids curriculum, focused on nutrition and childhood obesity, and was developmentally geared toward kids with strategic engagement of caregivers. *Ninos Saludable* eventually developed into *Movimiento Saludable* (Healthy Movement) for adolescents and continues as a component of the *Conexiones* Program.

Youth Health Prevention & Early Intervention

Latino youth are a unique subgroup who present some very troubling statistics in comparison to their adolescent counterparts. The general teen birth rate declined an astounding 33% in the nineties, perhaps due to the push for comprehensive sexual health education, but it remained steady for Latinos who now have the highest teen birth rate of any group in America (Child Trends, 2008). Mental health, particularly suicide attempts, is another alarming area where Latino teens consistently surpass their counterparts, with 15% of Latina girls attempting suicide, compared to 10% of White and Black teen girls (Centers for Disease Control, 2008).

Conexiones is a youth health prevention and early intervention program that targets some of the most concerning health and social issues facing Latino youth today. The program teaches youth about sexual health, dating violence, behavioral health including substance use and abuse and mental health, general nutrition, and overall well-being. The program brings together three main evidence-based curricula, Be Proud! Be Responsible!, developed by University of Pennsylvania researchers Loretta Sweet Jemmott, PhD, RN, FAAN, John B. Jemmott III, PhD, and Konstance A. McCaffree, PhD (1989); the Keepin' it REAL (Refuse, Explain, Avoid, Leave) curriculum, developed by Michael Hecht, PhD, and Flavio Francisco Marsiglia, PhD, from Penn State and Arizona State Universities, respectively (1989); and JARS, Justice, Accountability, Responsibility, Safety, a curriculum developed by the Pennsylvania Coalition Against Domestic Violence (2006).

Using these curricula, participants learn to apply skills in different settings and contexts including negotiation, resistance, and refusal skills. Screening tools used creatively within the group screen for dating violence, substance abuse, and mental health problems, and youth are encouraged to get tested for HIV. Youth are referred as needed to Congreso's programs addressing these areas. Nutrition is taught in serving and discussing healthy snacks that are often new to the participants, including fruit smoothies and guacamole. Participants are encouraged to learn more about their health by participating in *Movimiento Saludable* (Healthy Movement). Program data and youth input continue to enhance this program, where approximately 30% of participants annually are identified to be in the clinical range for mental health problems, 15% at high risk for substance abuse, and 17% as experiencing domestic violence. All identified youth are connected to services or, for those who are hesitant, continue to be encouraged to utilize services by *Conexiones* program staff or host case management staff for youth served in case management programs within the agency. A waiting list for each module speaks to the participants' receptivity to *Movimiento Saludable*.

Integrating Mental Health

As a major intervening and presenting variable across all of these programs, mental health has been formally integrated into many of Congreso's program models, particularly in the areas of women's and family health. Mental health problems present fairly pervasively among many health and social program clients, but particularly among Latinos. Although mental health problems and their causes vary dramatically, Latinos have significantly higher incidence rates. Latino teens are consistently much more likely than their Black and White classmates to attempt suicide, according to the Centers for Disease Control (2008), and adult Puerto Ricans, who comprise 66% of Philadelphia's Latinos, have the highest prevalence rate of psychiatric disorders among all Latino subgroups, according to a recent study published by the *American Journal of Public Health* (2007), titled "Prevalence of Psychiatric Disorders Across Latino Subgroups in the United States." Mental health problems are compounded by a significant underutilization of mental health care, as a result of stigma in the community and lack of availability of culturally competent, quality services.

For these reasons, mental health has been programmatically integrated into Congreso's family health programs, normalizing the need for and availability of services. Women are screened upon entry into social service programs using a variety of clinical screening instruments, including the Edinburgh Postnatal Depression Scale, the Youth Self-Report (YSR), and the Family Adaptability and Cohesion Evaluation Scale (FACES). Data is used by clinicians to educate on and normalize mental health and encourage treatment. For family health home visiting programs targeting adolescent and adult parents, mental health services are offered in the home for a mix of home and office-based treatment where clinicians and case managers work as a team. Women are encouraged to participate in clinical groups, such as a TREM group that uses the Trauma Recovery Empowerment Model developed by Maxine Harris. Appropriate participants are referred to the domestic violence program for structural family therapy with non-offending caregivers and children. Structural family therapy (SFT) began in the late 1960s in the Philadelphia Child Guidance Clinic under Dr. Salvadore Minuchin, beginning with urban Latino and African American families. Today, after much success, evidence and replication, SFT, with its holistic eco-structural approach, is a leading model for clinical work with Latino families.

For youth completing the YSR at the initiation of clinical services and again at 6–12 months, all participants dropped below the clinical range at follow-up, from a mean score of 61.67 to a score of 50 on internalizing behaviors. Participants completing the Edinburgh Depression Scale dropped from a mean score of 17.85 at pre-test to 9.95 at post-test, where a score of 9–15 indicates moderate depression and a score above 24 indicates severe depression. The FACES Inventory administered to each member in the family served through structural family therapy to assess family communication, family cohesion, and family satisfaction revealed a pre/post average increase of 13, 6, and 9 points respectively at post assessment. These data and strong show rates highlight the potential of services with mental health integration.

HIV Prevention

One final model deserving attention focuses on the power of peer support networks in preventing the spread of HIV. According to the Centers for Disease Control and Prevention, Latinos made up nearly 15% of the U.S. population in 2006, yet accounted for 19% of the diagnosed AIDS cases. Intravenous drug use (IDU) remains the second most prevalent mode of infection among Latinos, with an estimated 23% of Hispanic male HIV cases and an estimated 28% of Latinas exposed to HIV through IDU (CDC, 2006). The power of peer influence is particularly high among Latinos, where the community is frequently insulated and traditional models of public health prevention have missed Latinos almost entirely. From 2003–2005, Congreso worked with the Centers for Disease Control to develop and pilot the Social Network Project (SNP), which utilizes HIV-positive volunteer recruiters to identify their high-risk associates for outreach. Volunteers were recruited, trained, and coached to identify and approach their sexual and drug partners, with incentives offered for assistance targeting high-risk individuals. Through this method, the HIV identification rate went from 2.41% through the traditional outreach and counseling and testing approach to 4.22% through the social network approach. This model proved tremendously efficient in the face of diminishing resources, seeking out those most at-risk for HIV and most likely to spread the virus. Today, the program employs this among a variety of methods.

Conclusion

The four program models presented above share key characteristics. They each utilize relationship-building and established trust to connect people to services, they utilize participant input and data to strengthen the models, and they were developed largely for and by Latinos. Each also relies on participant information sharing and peer influence, and contributes to the public health education of the community. It is important to note that, while advances and improvements in overall American public health have much to do with the public health movements of the last fifty years or so, Latinos have largely been missed by these movements. Latinos have not had the focus and saturation, either in their countries of origin or here in the United States, where few public health campaigns have been truly tailored to this population. Just like boys and girls are different and require different interventions, so too are Latinos and other racial and ethnic groups. Much more research is needed to understand why many health disparities persist among Latinos, particularly when health outcomes do not mirror those in their countries of origin. And the power of the Spanish media in raising awareness, using tailored messages, must be recognized. While so much work remains, a great deal of success has been achieved within programs across the country that are ripe for replication.

12

Mental Health Services in Wellness Centers

Donna L. Torrisi, MSN, CRNP

Penny Killian, MSN, RN, PNP

Roberta Waite, EdD, RN, PMHCNS-BC

The World Health Organization states that there is not one "official" or "universal" definition of mental health. Individuals' mental health is affected by their culture and the cultures around them, as well as their subjective assessment and "emotional" well-being. When individuals use the term "mental health," they are most likely describing either a level of cognitive or emotional well-being or the absence of a mental health disorder. Emotional wellness, demonstrated by the overall comfort with and acceptance of one's full range of feelings, can be included within this viewpoint as well.

Nursing centers can provide individual and community support that allows for identification and support of good mental health among its clients and staff. These centers can provide a safe environment and trusting relationships, as well as places where patients have the ability to discuss and relate to issues that affect mental health. The organizations in the National Nursing Centers Consortium (NNCC) understand the importance of supporting clients and staff by encouraging their positive attitudes and attending to their emotional well-being, the capacity to live a full life, and the flexibility to deal with life's inevitable challenges.

An example of a wellness model developed by Myers, Sweeny, and Witmer (2000) includes five life tasks: essence or spirituality, work and leisure, friendship, love, and self-direction. The model outlines twelve sub-tasks that are identified as characteristics of healthy functioning and major components of wellness. These sub-tasks are: sense of worth, sense of control, realistic beliefs, emotional awareness and coping, problem solving and creativity, sense of humor, nutrition, exercise, self care, stress management, gender identity, and cultural identity. Personal development related to these tasks provides the means for a person to respond to the circumstances of life in a manner that promotes healthy functioning. While supporting this personal development may not be the *intended* focus of many nursing centers, when they are identified as Wellness Centers, their focus often encompasses many of these components. This serves to enhance clients' outcomes and provide opportunities for early identification and treatment of mental illness.

In maintaining good mental health, a positive attitude, high self-esteem, and a strong self-image are valuable attributes that support mentally healthy life experiences. Having available health care services that maintain an environment conducive to mental health wellness is a positive step to enhancing overall wellness.

Profiled in Appendix B are nursing centers that identify mental health wellness and prevention as a key component of their missions. While the way they work to accomplish this with their diverse populations may differ, the intentionality of their work crosses all of the organizations listed.

INTEGRATED BEHAVIORAL HEALTH SERVICES IN ONE HEALTH AND WELLNESS CENTER

Introduction and Background

In one Philadelphia Nurse Managed Health Center, the Family Practice & Counseling Network (FPCN), a behavioral health therapist is embedded into the primary care team in an attempt to provide immediate access for patients in distress and to address mental health crises, as well as chronic unstable problems. This has been done because the Network's traditional behavioral health services, although co-located within the health center sites, have almost always had a waiting list that precluded patients obtaining access when they most needed it. By the time a patient's name came to the top of the waiting list, the crisis had often passed. Sometimes the waiting list was so long that patients were referred to other behavioral health providers, but subsequent follow-up indicated that they often did not follow through with these referrals. Patients clearly prefer to receive their care in a familiar setting, so another reason for embedding a therapist in primary care is that many patients are resistant to obtaining care in a behavioral health department because of the stigma attached to mental illness and treatment.

In addition to being a Nurse Managed Health Center, the FPCN is also a Federally Qualified Health Center and a public housing grantee through the HRSA Bureau of Primary Health Care. The first FPCN center opened in July 1992 in a large public housing development. Today, there are three sites serving more than 10,000 patients from multiple public housing communities and surrounding low-income neighborhoods. Services include primary care, behavioral health care, dental services, and numerous health education programs for youth, individuals and families, and support programs for people living with cancer, HIV, and other chronic illnesses.

The FPCN has struggled since its inception to meet the behavioral health needs of the community, expanding the behavioral health department rapidly. Even with six or eight behavioral health therapists in each site providing traditional co-located care, the Network still could not meet the multiple and complex needs of all of its patients. Recognizing that there is a growing movement to integrate mental health and physical health in the primary care setting, the integrated model was introduced into one office to test its efficacy. Patients and primary care clinicians were so satisfied with the model that, within the next year, the model was spread to the other two sites.

Incidence of Depression

Mental illness is the second leading cause of disability and premature death (United States Department of Health and Human Services, 1999), second only to cardiovascular disease. One of the most prominent and devastating of the mental illnesses is depression, which has a one-year prevalence rate of 5–6 percent (Institute for Health Improvement, 2002). About 15% of the general population will suffer from Major Depressive Disorder sometime in their life, experiencing intense mental, emotional, and physical anguish and, often, substantial disability (Depression Guideline Panel, 1993). Twenty to forty percent of patients with diabetes or cardiac disease have major depression and depressed patients visit primary care providers three times more often than patients who are not depressed (Cole, S., & Cole, M. R., 2002). Diabetics who are also depressed have a higher level of non-adherence to their medical regime, an increase in HbA1c levels, and an increase in retinopathy, neuropathy, nephropathy, and macrovascular complications (DeGroot, Anderson, Freeland, Clouse & Lustman, 2001). Depression worsens health outcomes for people with medical illness and the existence of medical illness predisposes one to depression. Conversely, patients who have a sense of mental well-being, hopefulness, and optimism about the future are more likely to follow a medical regime and suffer less morbidity.

Women are at particular risk for depression, as are disadvantaged and low-income populations. While 15% of the general population will suffer from depression, studies of low-income urban women have shown a 40–50% rate of depressive symptoms (Lyons-Ruth, Connell, Grunebaum, & Botein, 1990). In a survey of adult patients completed by the National Nursing Centers Consortium, 38–40% of adult patients who received primary health care from their member centers in southeastern Pennsylvania reported symptoms of depression (National Nursing Centers Consortium, 2000). Eighty-six percent of FPCN's adult patients are female. A survey of FPCN adult patients noted a 20% incidence of depression and even higher for adults suffering with a chronic illness such as diabetes.

For people who are poor, signs of depression may be difficult to recognize. When someone in the middle class becomes depressed, his or her withdrawal or decreased capacity to function is usually obvious. However, for a poor person who may never have held a job or whose life is usually lacking in quality or productivity, symptoms of depression may not outwardly represent a significant change. In addition, someone whose life has always lacked joy may see their depressive state as "normal" and believe that everyone feels the way they feel.

Barriers to Treatment

There is a tremendous gap between the need for behavioral health services and their availability and accessibility of services to disadvantaged and minority populations, leaving a significant number of disadvantaged individuals untreated and trapped by their despair. Depression care in the United States is more fragmented than care of other chronic illnesses, creating a major gap between the recommended guidelines for care and actual care. It is estimated that only 19% of people with depression (fewer than one in five people) who see their primary care provider receive appropriate, guideline-based care (Institute for Health Improvement, 2002). In addition to a lack of availability of services, barriers to treatment that exist for disadvantaged groups, particularly women, include poverty, lack of health insurance, and lack of transportation and/or child care, as well as the stigma and shame attached to receiving behavioral health services (Hauenstein, 1996). For many people, mental health problems are synonymous with "being crazy" or weak, and patients believe that, by trying harder, they can will away or pray away mental health problems. There is a mistrust of medications and a fear that they are habit-forming or will make one look or feel like a "zombie." FPCN patients commonly list these reasons for their reluctance or refusal to accept medication or seek behavioral health therapy. Others agree to take medication or accept a behavioral health referral, appearing to go along because they do not want to counter their primary care provider's advice, but then never take the medication or show up for their therapy appointment.

Another barrier to treatment is the collusion of families who promote shame associated with a mental illness diagnosis and deny that problems are real. Collusion is especially common and destructive when there are family secrets, such as sexual abuse or incest. Many adult patients suffering with depression describe sexual abuse as a child and note that their parent cut any therapy short after one or two visits, telling the child or teen that it was not necessary. The depression returns in adulthood and is often associated with PTSD (post-traumatic stress disorder). An additional barrier lies in the fact that the lives of many patients who live in poverty are stressful and chaotic and they function in the moment and respond to crises rather than acting in a proactive and preventive manner.

Though the FPCN nurse-practitioners routinely screen for depression, they have often been left with a patient they know to be depressed who has neither the resources, the access, nor the will to obtain the behavioral health services they need. Though FPCN has expanded its behavioral health department to the maximum possible in response to the need and to the request of the

Philadelphia Office of Behavioral Health, there are never enough therapists to meet the needs of the population served.

Behavioral Health Integration Project

The FPCN health centers are each located in a low-income area of Philadelphia where issues of stress, anxiety, abuse, depression, chronic health problems, and PTSD abound. To meet the needs of its patients, the FPCN has integrated a behavioral health therapist into the primary care team in each of its three health center sites. The Network funds these therapists through multiple private grants and with reimbursements obtained through billing third party payers, primarily Medicaid and Medicare. The consultant's role is to provide support and assistance to both primary care providers and their patients without engaging in extended specialty behavioral health care. The model and associated interventions, which have strong empirical support, rely heavily on cognitive-behavioral theory because they are problem-focused assessments, which can be implemented quickly using handouts and other instructional aids. The emphasis is on support and behavior change and the goal is improved function and quality of life.

The behavioral health providers support improved detection of depression, anxiety, and other mental health issues through universal screening by primary care providers who use targeted questions to screen for depression and other issues such as abuse. If there is a positive response to any of the questions, the nine-question prime MD tool, may be used to gain additional information regarding the patient's mood to pass on to the behavioral health therapist. In addition to screening for depression, nurse practitioners ask other questions to elicit indication of psychosocial problems. Primary providers are more likely to discuss mental health issues with patients when there is a therapist available to help manage problems should they surface. Examples of queries include:

- Everyone experiences stress in their lives to some degree, how are you currently managing the stress in your life?
- How are things going at work?
- Is anyone treating you in an abusive manner, physically or mentally?
- Are you having any problems with mood swings?
- How are your children doing?
- How are you sleeping?
- How is your appetite?
- What do you do for pleasure?
- Are you having any trouble with feeling lonely or isolated?
- Who do you usually turn to for support when you are having a problem?

If a patient gives any hints about depression, anxiety, or stress, the provider might simply say, "Can you tell me more about that?" When a problem surfaces, the patient is asked permission to introduce another member of the primary care team. The behavioral health therapist introduces himself or herself to the patient as a therapist and spends time with the patient in the exam room, either alone or in the presence of the nurse practitioner. The behavioral health provider's intervention is brief, 15–30 minutes, half the time of a usual visit and requires only the documentation of a progress note compared to a four-hour intake required by the traditional behavioral health Medicaid insurer.

For this model, FPCN has committed to physically not separating the behavioral health provider from the rest of the primary care process. In fact, the behavioral health provider shares the same office space (called the touch down room) as the primary care providers. In this system, behavioral health is not a specialty service, but rather a routine component of medical care. A patient is just as likely to see a behavioral health provider as any other member of the primary care team. The behavioral health provider records progress notes in the health center's electronic medical record, which the FPCN has been using for almost three years, so documentation is also integrated.

Literature shows that there is a strong relationship between psychological distress and medical utilization and that the integration model of primary care and behavioral health has a positive impact on reducing medical utilization and improving patient functioning. The improved outcomes of the integrated model include more satisfied patients and providers and lower total health costs. Most importantly, the model addresses some of the barriers to care, such as access and shame associated with entering the behavioral health department, because the care is provided within the primary care department, right in the exam room. The patient may present with depression or anxiety or, more commonly, with frequent somatic symptoms such as back pain, bad nerves, stomach aches, or headaches. The primary care provider makes a referral upon determining that there is no medical pathology to explain the symptoms. The therapist provides almost immediate attention to the patient upon receiving a referral from the primary care provider. The patient perceives the care received from the behavioral health therapist as part of their primary care experience, so the patient not only receives the needed service, but also does not have to confront the stigma, inconvenience, and lack of access to a behavioral health program.

Case Studies

■ A patient suffering from depression related to the loss of a spouse was immediately referred for support and development of coping skills. The patient was also provided with educational material on depression, grief and loss, bereavement groups, and stress reduction tools. Since the patient was believed to be clinically depressed, the behavioral health therapist discussed medication with her and her nurse practitioner. The patient's behavioral health goals were recorded in the medical chart, so that coping strategies were reinforced during routine medical visits. In this case, the behavioral health therapist set up a follow-up appointment with the patient separate from the primary care visit. (In this model, the patient is typically seen from one to three visits.)

■ A fourteen-year-old teen boy was seen with his mother. She noted that he had become withdrawn and depressed following an incident where a teen girl was aggressive and touched him inappropriately at a family gathering. The boy and his mother spent thirty minutes with the therapist and after the one session he was able to move on and return to his usual demeanor.

▪ A woman suffering from post-partum depression was seen for a brief consult and two additional sessions, after which time she was feeling better. The therapist provided her with validation and a biochemical understanding of symptoms and helped her develop a support team within her family until she recovered.

▪ A 68-year-old female with diabetes had stopped taking her medication because she was overwhelmed and stressed regarding the care of her spouse who had Alzheimer's disease and she was grieving his loss. The therapist provided her with support, referred her to a women's depression group, and assured she had resources to help with her spouse. The woman began taking her medications again and got her diabetes back under control.

The therapist uses a "behavioral prescription" pad to record the plan and any follow-up appointment time and gives it to the patient. Communication back to the primary care provider is one of the therapist's highest priorities, often requiring the therapist to stay late to have a face-to-face conversation so that feedback is given the same day the patient is seen and allowing the primary care provider and the behavioral health provider to best support the patient in recovering from depression. At the primary care level, preventing another occurrence of depression takes on the same importance as assuring the patient's general health. The advantages of a fully integrated approach are better coordination of care, better clinical outcomes, reduced medical practice costs, and increased customer satisfaction. Most importantly, practicing side by side allows primary care and behavioral health providers to learn from each other and form a thorough appreciation of the interdependence of the body and the mind. Patients deemed to have more severe or chronic mental illness may be referred to the behavioral health department for traditional psychotherapy. By utilizing the integrated brief therapy model, fewer patients overall are referred to the behavioral health department, thus decreasing the wait time for patients who really need the intensive treatment.

Sustainability

The behavioral health clinician is able to bill Community Behavioral Health, Philadelphia's Medicaid insurer, so this model will become self-supporting. An FQHC is permitted to bill for a primary care and a behavioral health visit on the same day. According to federal regulation under the Prospective Payment System, the FQHC must be reimbursed at their cost. Patients who are uninsured are not charged a fee in addition to the primary care fee they paid, but may be charged a nominal fee for a visit if they return to see the behavioral therapist for follow-up. FPCN has noticed that this cutting edge model is of great interest to potential funders, including corporations and foundations.

Resources

Action Planning for Prevention and Recovery A Self-Help Guide. http://mentalhealth.samhsa.gov/publications/allpubs/SMA-3720/developing.asp

A portal to the Web sites of a number of multi-agency health initiatives and activities of the U.S. Department of Health and Human Services and other Federal departments and agencies. http://www.health.gov

Bright Futures (tool kit). http://www.brightfutures.org/georgetown.html

Developing a Recovery and Wellness Lifestyle A Self-Help Guide. http://mentalhealth.samhsa.gov/publications/allpubs/SMA-3718/default.asp

Dedicated to those interested in managing stress, maximizing performance and enhancing emotional health. http://www.OptimalHealthConcepts.com/Stress

International Council of Nurses (best practices guidelines). http://www.icn.ch/guidelines.htm

Mental Health Matters. http://www.mental-health-matters.com/

National Institute of Mental Health. www.nimh.nih.gov/

Pocket Guide to Mental Health Resources. SAMHSA'S National Mental Health Information Center: Center for Mental Health Resources. http://mentalhealth.samhsa.gov/publications/allpubs/SMA01-3509/Default.asp

Wellness Information Zone. Information on diseases and conditions, healthy lifestyles, local health resources and navigating the health system sponsored by the Humana foundation. http://www.wellzone.org

IV

Student
Learning

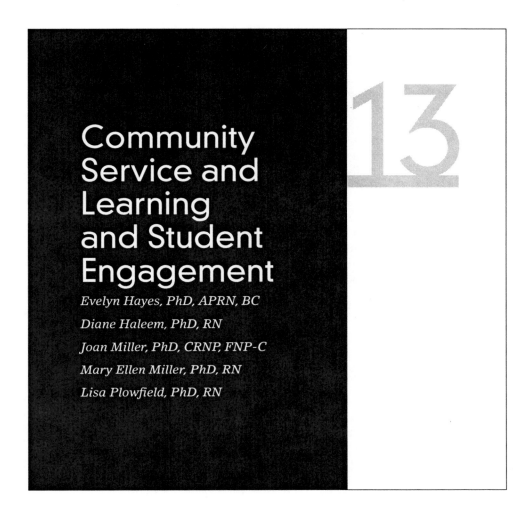

Community Service and Learning and Student Engagement

Evelyn Hayes, PhD, APRN, BC

Diane Haleem, PhD, RN

Joan Miller, PhD, CRNP, FNP-C

Mary Ellen Miller, PhD, RN

Lisa Plowfield, PhD, RN

"When I thought about the homeless, I always thought of a man sitting on a street vent. I now know that many families with children are homeless and use local soup kitchens. This service experience has really made me aware of who the homeless are and what needs they have."

Introduction

Community Service and Learning (CSL) is defined as a teaching and learning strategy that integrates meaningful community service, instruction, and reflection, to enrich the learning experience, teach civic responsibility, and strengthen communities (National Service Learning Clearinghouse, 2008). The "service" and the "learning" components are equal. Each component enhances the other and no component holds greater weight (Sigmon, 1994).

The Corporation for National and Community Service cites Eyler and Giles (1999) who suggest several characteristics of CSL:

- Supporting learning through active participation in service experiences;
- Promoting cooperation rather than competition and thus providing teamwork;
- Providing an opportunity for students to use skills and knowledge in real-life situations;
- Extending learning beyond the classroom and into the community; and
- Providing of structured time for students to reflect by thinking, discussing, and validating their experiences (Miller & Giugliano, 2006).

CSL provides opportunities for students to partner with key community agencies to help meet the needs of underserved and vulnerable populations. Benefits for students include academic growth, life skill development, and civic engagement (Astin & Sax, 1998). In addition, service learning enhances the critical thinking skills of students as they engage in problem solving with community partners (Sedlak, Doheny, Panthofer, & Anaya, 2003). Broader implications of service learning include interpersonal, social, and moral development, as well as increased awareness of community, national, and global problems, as noted by the student quoted above.

Contemporary students must have the opportunity to look beyond the narrow boundaries of their own life experiences. Community service learning provides a venue to prepare students for progressive leadership in the community. This requires more than fleeting service experiences. It also requires partnerships that are borne of mutual interest and commitment to both students' growth and the community's ability to meet its own goals. The purpose of incorporating a CSL component into the nursing curriculum is to provide a *legitimate* experience, whereby students apply theoretical content to a community setting (Miller & Giugliano, 2006).

A distinction must be made between service learning that is integrated into the curriculum, and for which credit is given, and not-for-credit or volunteer activity. Volunteerism is usually associated with performance of a service out of interest in doing for others. For example, students may visit elderly residents in a nursing home to relieve the isolation residents often experience. As students learn about the health experiences of the elderly, they may seek more structured experiences in the care of the elderly. Interest generated through volunteer activity may prompt service learning projects for which credit may or may not be awarded. Both volunteer and course-related services have value in promoting the professional development of student nurses. Additionally, volunteerism does not contain a formal reflective activity post event. Reflection is a hallmark of CSL.

Overview of Community Service Learning in the Health Professions

In a review of literature, Champagne (2006) outlines the origin and evolution of service learning in the health professions. According to Champagne (2006), Sigmon (1979) defined service learning as a reciprocal process. Community members define their needs and service providers define what is to be learned through service. The outcome is empowerment of the community to care for its own needs. Champagne (2006) summarizes Polvika's (1995) model for service learning. Polvika stressed the need to address environmental, situational, and partnership-building issues when establishing interagency relationships. Environmental issues include socioeconomic and political factors. Situational issues include resources available to partnering agencies and the goals and tasks associated with a collaborative project. Prior to the initiation of a project, partnering agencies involved must address staffing issues, flow of information, and terms of evaluation. Foss, Bonaiuto, Johnson, and Moreland (2003) modified Polvika's model for interagency relationships and developed a conceptual model to guide a collaborative nursing program and community partnership. The model addresses pre-partnership conditions, principles of partnerships, and concepts to guide assessment of partnership outcomes. Pre-partnership conditions included examination of the roles of each partner, terms of the relationship, and steps to take to ensure mutual benefit. Partnerships are more likely to be successful when principles of partnership, such as shared mission, mutual trust, and open communication, are honored. Similarly, outcomes are more likely to be positive when partners respond to needed change and share credit for success.

Butin (2003) describes criteria essential for integration of service learning into education. These include respect, reciprocity, relevance, and reflection. Service learning projects must demonstrate respect for partner agencies and the populations served. The providers and the recipients of service must both engage in the planning process. At the same time, service learning projects must be relevant to course objectives and students must engage in reflection on the benefits of service learning from theoretical, personal, and community perspectives (Table 13.1). Thorough evaluation of service learning partnerships is essential to ensure justification for future programming.

CSL and the Nursing Process

The approach to CSL follows the nursing process, and thus is well suited to nursing education and projects in wellness centers. *Assessment* of the needs of the service organization and the population is the first step. Assessment helps

13.1 Somatic Complaints Questions

SERVICE-learning	SERVICE-LEARNING
Intensive service project	Intensive service project
Loosely linked to learning; often a reflective course component.	Central to coursework; highly integrated reflective component
Service-learning	service-LEARNING
Moderate to low intensity	Moderate to low intensity
Service Project	Service Project
Add-on or optional service project. Loosely linked with course content.	Reflection on community-based experience tightly linked with course content. Students apply academic theory to community situation.

X axis: Degree of explicit educational linkages between theory and practice in assignments, classroom, exams, papers, etc.
Y axis: Degree of service requirements in the course
©Nadinne Cruz Service-Learning Matrix Exercise
Adapted from Sigmon (1994)

in both identifying and *planning* the CSL activity. Developing objectives for the service-learning project facilitates the *implementation* and execution of the CSL activities. Implementation can be done in one period of service activity, a few occasions of service activity, or over an extended period of time, such as an entire semester. After the service is completed, *evaluation* of effectiveness is important. Getting the viewpoint (both quantitative and qualitative) from all involved parties, including the participants, agency representatives, and self (the student nurse) help determine the effectiveness and value of the CSL activity.

Adding Value to Nursing Wellness Centers

Most nurses enter the profession wanting to care well for others. Novice nurses experience excitement and passion for the work they have chosen, often at an early age. Many enter the profession with confidence, poise, respect for authority, and the capacity to work well in teams. As Patton (2007) states, the new generation of nurses holds promise for the future of the profession. Through mentoring, coaching, and role modeling, experienced nurses can foster the professional growth of the new professional nurse.

The American Association of Colleges of Nursing (AACN) (2008) has identified the following core values as essential to professional development of the nurse and the welfare of patients: altruism, autonomy, human dignity, integrity, and social justice. Nursing wellness centers provide an environment where the core values of the nursing profession can be modeled. Nursing wellness centers traditionally provide care and programs for underserved and vulnerable populations. In such settings, the core values of the nursing profession can be integrated into academic education. Nursing students need exposure to core professional values, as well as psychomotor skills (Shaw & Degazon, 2008). Students for whom core values were integrated into the curriculum reported greater ease during the socialization process as they entered the profession. Based on the work of Shaw and Degazon, each value can be defined and examined in light of integrative strategies for learning in a wellness center environment.

Altruism: Altruism refers to a selfless concern for the welfare of others. Faculty can model altruism by providing support for students and encouraging students to develop caring relationships with one another, staff, and the patients they serve. In a culture of caring in a wellness center, students will more likely be able to work with patients who may be different from themselves. Students often find working with the underprivileged rewarding. They gain a sense of the difference they can make in the lives of others. Reflective journaling may be one strategy to capture the meaning of what is required to care selflessly for others.

Autonomy: Autonomy refers to self-determination and direction. In a nursing wellness center, faculty and students often partner to make independent decisions or assist others to make decisions about their own care. Students encounter cultural differences related to health care in wellness centers. Faculty can model respect for the autonomy of patients whose cultural values may differ from students and other health professionals. Post-conference discussion or writing exercises regarding the challenges associated with offering support for another's values when different from one's own may strengthen the capacity of the student nurse to respect the right for self-determination in matters of health.

Human Dignity: Human dignity involves having respect for the individual worth and unique qualities of others. Students encounter individuals with differing values, ethnic background, and lifestyles when working in nursing wellness centers. When faculty model respect for all who present in a wellness center, students are more likely to overcome prejudices and develop a non-prejudicial approach to nursing care.

Integrity: Integrity involves acting according to one's own values and the highest standards of the profession. Faculty can model excellence for students in nursing wellness centers. They can also model advocacy so that students learn they can serve as agents of change when policies and rules in an environment limit the quality of care a person should receive. Focused discussion, reflective writing, and review of standards of practice can reinforce the importance of personal and professional values.

Social Justice: Social justice refers to fair and equitable distribution of resources. When students work with faculty in nursing wellness centers, they encounter multiple situations that raise concern about the community needs and interests. Observance of local government practices and participation in health conferences and events with more senior faculty may contribute to the development of heightened awareness of social justice issues.

Nurse-managed wellness centers can provide exposure to diverse populations and a variety of health-related issues for prospective students and those already enrolled in nursing programs. Faculty serve as mentors, coaches, and role models as they seek to create a caring culture, one based on the core values of the nursing profession. It is essential that experienced nurses create a value-focused culture that will foster development of the desire to care well for others among student and novice nurses.

Benefits of Service Learning

The benefits of CSL activities extend beyond the community and/or the agency in which the service is performed. Faculty and students also both benefit from CSL activities. Benefits of CSL for faculty include an expanded role, enhanced teaching and learning, and the opportunity to link an academic area of interest with unmet community needs. As faculty advance their areas of research interest, they function as mentors or role models, providing direction and guidance for students aspiring to become responsible professionals. Benefits of building CSL into required nursing curriculum include long-term sustainability of services in the community, lowering the cost and funding needed for services, faculty buy-in and support of services, and increased manpower available to become involved with the community. Despite these benefits, faculty members frequently cite time constraints, lack of recognition, and lack of institutional support as barriers to faculty involvement. Several authors suggest linking CSL projects to the teaching effectiveness and research interests of faculty (Harrington, 1999; Eyler, Giles, Stenson, & Gray, 2001; Cushman, 2002). Steinke and Fitch (2007) indicate that the quality and quantity of CSL assessments need to be increased and conclude that, as assessments of CSL are further developed, faculty can present their work at conferences related to the scholarship of teaching and learning, thereby stimulating more service-learning researchers and research tools.

Students report multiple benefits associated with participation in CSL projects. CSL exposes students to vulnerable populations and to the needs of targeted communities served by wellness centers (i.e., the homeless, Hispanic, older adults). CSL also increases students' future intent to perform service in their own communities post-graduation (reported via student evaluations and anecdotes). Reinforcement of classroom learning, greater awareness of community needs, increased social responsibility, and sensitivity to moral issues were among the benefits reported by students involved in a program designed to help teen parents transition to parenthood (Bentley & Ellison, 2005). Sedlak et al. (2003) indicate that enhanced critical thinking is also a benefit of service learning. Students also develop a sense of community that extends beyond classroom and clinical experiences.

When accompanied by the use of reflective journaling, service learning contributes to the professional development of students (Sedlak et al., 2003). Structured reflection reinforces the learning that takes place in the community setting. No matter what form the reflection activity takes, it is imperative that instructors ask students about their personal lessons learned along the way, as well as the challenges they encountered during the CSL activity. Students have often reported initial feelings of frustration and sometimes even dismay, but over time have shifted their focus to the mutual benefits revealed to both the student and the recipients of the service activity (Miller & Guiglano, 2006).

Challenges Associated With Community Service and Learning

In addition to the benefits noted above, both students and faculty cite challenges associated with service learning. Students cite increased time required in the preparation for teaching and evaluation materials included in service learning experiences. Faculty note that scheduling, reviewing journals, and evaluation procedures constitute an added burden associated with incorporating service learning experiences into the curriculum. Integrating service, research, and scholarship may be one way to generate greater interest in service learning among faculty.

Implementation of Community Service and Learning

When incorporating CSL activities into the curriculum, course syllabi must specifically state that CSL is among the course requirements. It is necessary that course objectives explicitly state expected outcomes related to the CSL component of the course. Objectives of a course involving CSL can include the following: knowledge, skill, attitudes/values, and service. An example of each category follows.

- Knowledge Objective: To define an organization that assists those who are having difficulty in obtaining health care services, its goals and objectives, its structure, its activities, its sources of support, and its impacts.
- Skill Objective: To demonstrate ability to use actual experiences to evaluate the adequacy of activities in elder centers.
- Attitude/Value/Commitment Objectives: To verbalize a commitment to use available opportunities to help those who are homeless.
- Service Objective: To provide assistance to an organization that is helping people who are homeless seek employment.

Having specified objectives will assist students in focusing their efforts and enrich their CSL experience.

Examples of Community Service and Learning Projects in Nursing Programs

Service learning is often utilized as an educational tool in nursing programs. CSL fits into the mission of schools of nursing and can be incorporated into clinical courses, such as Obstetrical, Pediatrics, Psychiatric Mental Health, Community/ Public Health, and Medical Surgical Nursing courses. When incorporated into the curriculum, the CSL project should be structured, monitored, and evaluated (Long, Larsen, Hussey, & Travis, 2001). The degree of structure may vary according to students' knowledge, clinical experience, and skill level.

Using a "wall-less" concept of a nursing wellness center, undergraduate and graduate nursing students can participate in CSL activities in a variety of community settings. The scope of student involvement increases as the complexity of the course-related material increases. Learning objectives for both students and community members or agencies served are defined prior to implementation of the CSL project. The degree of supervision and oversight required varies according to the knowledge and skill level of the students and the degree of risk for harm for either the students or care recipients, as well as educational institution and agency regulations. Examples of how CSL can be implemented across the curriculum are found in Table 13.2.

13.2 CSL Implementation

Course	Student	Target Population	CSL Activity	Implementation Site
Foundations of Nursing	Undergraduate Sophomore	Adult females	Client interviews and arts and crafts projects	Women's ceramics class
Pharmacology	Undergraduate Sophomore	Elderly	Brown bag lunch for medication review	Senior Center
Pediatrics	Undergraduate Sophomore	Elementary school age	Homework tutoring and reading assistance	After-school program
Disease Management	Undergraduate Junior	Elderly	Social support via game activities incorporating health education	Senior citizen apartment complex
Chronic Illness	Undergraduate Junior	Homeless adults	Foot inspections and foot soaks	Soup kitchen
Public Health	Undergraduate Senior	All ages	Primary and secondary prevention activities at Community Health Fairs	Various community sites
Public Health	Graduate	Adolescents and families	Comprehensive needs assessment and interactive communication workshops	University setting

Evaluation of Community Service and Learning Activities

Faculty, students, and agency personnel all participate in the evaluation of CSL projects and their outcomes. Long et al. (2001) address the need for both formative and summative evaluation of service learning projects. Formative evaluation is often required when a project is ongoing and involving incremental knowledge development. This type of evaluation is often used in projects that take place over time. Summative evaluation is usually conducted upon the completion of a project to determine if learning objectives were met. For example, if a community assessment and health fair project occurs over a full semester, both formative and summative evaluations should be performed to evaluate the effectiveness of the project.

In the CSL examples presented in Table 13.2, summative evaluations were conducted following the sophomore and junior level projects to determine if learning objectives of both students and community members were met. Sophomore students reported that their CSL projects helped them overcome the "fear they had about going out into the community." All levels of student, undergraduate and graduate, remarked that they were encouraged by the knowledge they had gained through their community experiences. They felt they had made a difference in the lives of those they served. They also stated that they enjoyed working as a team to plan and implement teaching modules and activities for their clients. The undergraduate students acknowledged the need to work on public speaking skills. Faculty benefits of these CSL projects cited included enriched teaching opportunities, increased engagement of students in the learning process, and greater awareness of community needs.

Student Reflections on Community Service and Learning Experiences

Student reflections usually occur in the form of narrative reflection papers. However, students should also be encouraged to perform their reflection activity in the manner that they personally find rewarding. In addition to narrative writing, artwork, poetry, creative posters, and other artistic forms of expression can be encouraged. In one University setting, undergraduate students performed CSL activities towards the end of the fall semester, close to the Christmas holiday season. A few students spent time at a local mall working at a kiosk that provided free gift-wrapping services. They combined their gift-wrapping hours with a visible poster presentation to the shoppers. Their poster highlighted nutritional tips on how to eat well and keep fit during the holiday season to avoid gaining the traditional five to ten holiday pounds. As their method of reflection, these students wrapped an extra large gift box with holiday paper and glued several large gift tags onto the box. The gift tags contained narrative statements describing their feelings regarding this CSL experience.

When analyzing student reflection papers post-CSL experience, several themes emerged. Some of these were:

> ▨ Teamwork: Students felt they were able to collaborate with the agency where they did their community service. They stated that partnerships were also formed with the participants whom they were helping. Students

that worked in teams also gained the experience of and valued collaborating and coordinating with a fellow nursing colleague.

- Leadership Role: Students took the initiative to determine what CSL project they were going to address by assessing the participants' needs, planning and developing the objectives and interventions, and evaluating the outcomes. They were able to organize meetings, prepare a program, and connect with the participants in a very meaningful way.
- Collaboration: Students collaborated with the agency, their faculty, the participants, and their fellow student colleagues, and found the experience to be meaningful.
- Embrace Difference/New Perspectives: Students expressed a better understanding of different cultures and life circumstances, i.e., Students cared for participants who were alcoholics, homeless, terminally ill, elderly, and participants with mental health challenges. Some examples of student statements follow:

"Hearing about the disease from a family member (of someone who has Alzheimer's) put everything into a whole new perspective."

"I gained great respect for the clients in their abilities to share their stories, fears, failures, and their choice to work hard to battle against their substance abuse."

"I gained a lot personally from this experience. I felt that many people think that aging is a time when older adults do not do anything. The seniors that I talked with at the Center were so open to learning: they wanted to hear what I had to say."

- Contributing: Students felt they made a difference in the lives of others. One student who did her service learning at an Alzheimer's Caregiver support group stated, "I would like to continue to attend and lend support to the support group."

It is important to note that, in addition to performing CSL experiences at sites served by Wellness Centers, students can also complete CSL activities at their own college. Senior students helped in a skills and health assessment class by posting and being available in the lab after class to help their student colleagues practice their skills. One student noted, "The students seemed to enjoy being helped and it was a pleasure to see them feel more confident about doing a physical assessment. Now, because I am more comfortable in performing that skill, it is useful to pass that skill on to others." Another student shared, "Teaching these skills helped me to realize just how much I learned over the past year and a half, so that was a big confidence booster for me."

University Community Service and Learning Committee

Many universities have a formalized Service Learning Committee comprised of faculty and staff from multiple schools within the university. Having a university-wide Service Learning Committee, addressing service learning needs and issues, can help coordinate information to support both the students and faculty. This is a tremendous step in preventing duplication of work by looking for community partners and resources. Having a mission statement, goals, and training can assist in the success of a Committee's function and vision (Mercer & Brungardt, 2007).

Fort Hays University recommends six steps when initiating a Service Learning Committee:

- Establish Committee members.
- Develop a definition, mission, and goals for service learning for the campus.
- Educate faculty about pedagogy and learning benefits of service learning.
- Generate enthusiasm among the student body.
- Educate the community at large, in participator community agencies, about service learning and the potential benefits to their agencies as well as to the broader community (Mercer & Brungardt, 2007).

Within the University CSL Committee, there can be subcommittees, which could consist of:

- Service Learning Handbook Development Committee
- Faculty Development Committee
- CSL Webpage Development Committee

The CSL Committee should meet regularly, either monthly or several times each semester. Meetings may consist of topical discussions, sharing of community resources, and ideas to strengthen syllabi. Some suggested topics of discussion include resources needed to support fellow faculty, a current list of partners in the community interested in collaboration, available resource Web links, book recommendations, library suggestions, and a list of faculty interested in co-curricular service learning projects.

Conclusion

Schools of Nursing and nurse-managed wellness centers are a "natural fit" to promote CSL activities with graduate and undergraduate students. Replication of an initiative, such as the "Neat Feet" project highlighted in Appendix D, is achievable. The following strategies are recommended as means to promote CSL and engaging students in Wellness Center activities:

- Deans and directors must be actively engaged in promoting CSL activities in undergraduate and graduate curricula.
- Wellness Center nursing staff should serve as adjunct faculty at Schools of Nursing.

- CSL activities should be incorporated into course syllabi.
- Faculty from nursing schools should collaborate with community service and learning departments/divisions on campus.
- Nursing faculty should get on group e-mail "listservs" for notification of funding opportunities for CSL activities.
- Coordinators of CSL at nursing schools can contact other coordinators of CSL activities on campus, and at other campuses in their locale, and hold "brown bag" lunches, where best practices can be shared.

When measures such as these are employed, successful CSL initiatives can occur that benefit students, faculty, and community participants. Helpful tools are found in Appendix D.14. All parties involved are transformed by CSL encounters. Service learning projects echo what we do as nurses, which is to partner with patients, families, and communities, in the context of their environment, to maximize health and well-being. Margaret Newman (2003) puts it best, "Nurses who partner with patients experience the joy of participating in the expanding process of others and find their own lives are enhanced and transformed."

Resources

Service Learning Links:
> www.servicelearning.org/
> www.servicelearning.org/what_is_service-learning/service-learning_is/index.php
> www.service-learningpartnership.org/
> www.newhorizons.org/strategies/service_learning/front_service.htm
> www.learnandserve.gov/
> www.islonline.org/
> www.compact.org
> http://wpcarey.asu.edu/csl/
> www.ipsl.org/

Service Learning Projects:
> www.marylandpublicschools.org/MSDE/programs/servicelearning/project_ideas
> www.mssa.sailorsite.net/ideas.html
> www.epa.gov/epaoswer/general/educate/svclearn.pdf

International Service Learning:
> www.islonline.org/
> www.ipsl.org/
> www.islonline.com/
> www.servicelearning.org/instant_info/hot_topics/international/index.php
> www.amizade.org/
> www.fiu.edu/~time4chg/Library/ideas.html

Service Learning Ideas:
> www.psc.disney.go.com/disneychannel/learningtoserve/resources/index.html
> www.marylandpublicschools.org/MSDE/programs/servicelearning/project_ideas
> www.paservicelearning.org/Project_Ideas/
> www.northern.edu/ASLP/Projects2.html

Benefits of Service Learning:
> www.servicelearning.org/lsa/bring_learning/

Service Learning Curriculum:
> www.learningindeed.org/tools/other/currnet.html
> www.cde.ca.gov/ci/cr/sl/
> www.education-world.com/a_curr/curr188.shtml
> www.aacc.nche.edu/.../Current/HorizonsServiceLearningProject/CurriculumTools/
> CurriculumTools.htm

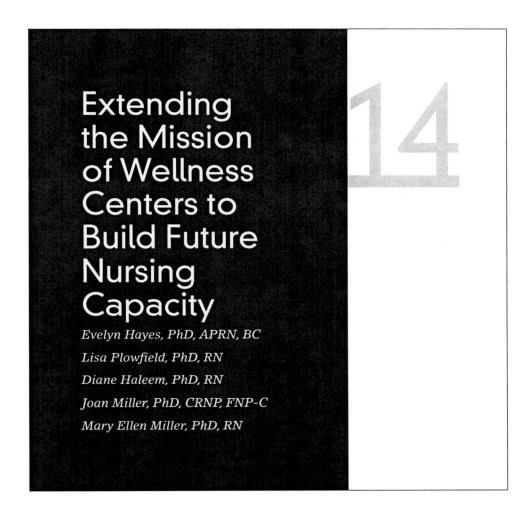

Extending the Mission of Wellness Centers to Build Future Nursing Capacity

14

Evelyn Hayes, PhD, APRN, BC

Lisa Plowfield, PhD, RN

Diane Haleem, PhD, RN

Joan Miller, PhD, CRNP, FNP-C

Mary Ellen Miller, PhD, RN

"The future starts today, not tomorrow."

Pope John Paul II

The Current Nursing Shortage

The U.S. health care workforce is in a vulnerable state. Nursing is a crucial component of the health care workforce. It is projected that, by the year 2016, more than 1.2 new and replacement nurses will be needed in the workforce for every current nurse (United States Department of Labor Statistics, 2007). There are an increasing number of registered nurses reaching "retirement age," which means there will be an increased need for people to consider nursing as a career option to replace them. The demand for nurses is expected to grow by 2% to 3% each year according to the American Association of College Nurses, using Dr. Peter Buerhaus' data from The Future of Nursing Workforce in the United States: Data, Trends and Implications (AACN, 2008). The nursing shortage is expected to reach 500,000 nurses by the year 2025. These are staggering numbers!

In addition to the shortage, data also show that the nurses currently caring for patients don't mirror the ethnic and cultural diverse backgrounds of their patients. There are 2,694,540 licensed registered nurses. Of these, approximately 87% of all RNs are Caucasian; 4.9% are African American; 3.7% are Asian or Pacific Islander; 2% are Hispanic; 0.5% are American Indian or Alaska Native; and 1.2% categorize themselves as "multiracial" (two or more races) (Minority Nurse.com, 2000). Approximately 146,902 RNs are men, totaling 5.4% of the total number of nurses. The average age of the RN population in the United States is 45.2 years. Only 9.1% of RNs are under the age of 30. Twenty-one percent of male RNs are 50 years of age or older, compared with 34% of female RNs (Minority Nurse.com, 2000). Increasing the number of boys and girls from all cultures and ethnic backgrounds who consider nursing as a career is a priority.

The *Kids Into Health Careers* Initiative

To address the current and ongoing predicted shortage of health care professionals, the Health Resources Service Administration (HRSA) Bureau of Health Professions has encouraged community-based organizations to develop linkages with teenage youth from diverse backgrounds. The objectives of this linkage were to inform and encourage minority and disadvantaged adolescents of educational and career opportunities in health professions and assist in preparing them for education in health care professions.

The federally funded *Kids Into Health Careers* (KIHC) program supports initiatives that focus on increasing the numbers of young girls and boys, including those from culturally diverse backgrounds, who consider nursing as their profession. The KIHC initiative has resulted in nursing centers establishing a wide variety of programs that have further extended the reach and original missions of wellness centers in this area.

The goals of the KIHC campaign, health career building for the future, are to:

- Inform students, parents, teachers, and guidance counselors about careers in the health professions;
- Create optimism about the value, rewards, and accessibility of health profession careers;
- Provide facts about the availability of financial aid for health professions training;
- Increase awareness about the need for under-represented minorities in health professions; and
- Improve overall access to health for under-represented minority and disadvantaged populations by increasing the minority applicant pool for health professions training.

The KIHC initiative is designed to reach a variety of stakeholders/constituents. Students, ages K-12, parents, guidance counselors, teachers, administrators, and other partners are the groups of focus for this initiative. The targeted populations are minority, under-represented, and potentially vulnerable children. KIHC is a way to build bridges to address diverse and complex health care needs within a population, as well as to reach out to under-represented groups to develop a more culturally competent workforce.

Example Program Initiatives

University of Delaware Nursing Center: "Picture Yourself a Nurse"

In the University of Delaware Nursing Center: "Picture Yourself a Nurse" project, guided by social cognition theory and the Healthy Cities framework, children from kindergarten through grade 12 were targeted. Social cognition theory dictated the use of fun activities, discussion with nurses, and free literature and photographs depicting oneself as a nurse, to bring nursing as a viable career option to the forefront of children's thoughts. The Healthy Cities framework promotes local grassroots initiatives in meeting the health and health care system needs of one's own community. Nursing faculty partnered with community agencies in this project to promote the consideration of nursing as a profession. This project was funded by US PHS grant #1D11HP00239-01.

"Will you help us care for tomorrow?" was a banner message to bring people to the exhibit. A "Kodak" moment program was designed, giving children a chance to stand behind plywood depictions of UD scrubs and nursing situations (holding ethnically diverse babies, wearing stethoscopes around their necks) and to take photos labeled with their name and "Tomorrow's Nurse/Future Nurse." Children, their parents, and friends waited patiently in lines to participate in this activity, which created an ideal opportunity for student nurses in professional attire to engage the youth and family/friends in discussion about health and health careers. Some children had little knowledge about nursing and the diverse career opportunities it offers. Parents consistently commented on the impact of the nursing shortage on health care. All participants were eager to learn more about nursing and viewed the nursing profession positively as a career choice. Young persons outside the targeted age group frequently requested to participate, including preschoolers and young adults. Even parents of babies requested to have their baby photographed as a nurse (Plowfield & Hayes, 2006).

Also through the project, nurses from the wellness center and nursing students acted as role models, recruiters, and ambassadors. Nursing students and faculty provided children in schools, as well as at health fairs and community events, the opportunity to be involved in age appropriate games and health promotion activities, and gave them colorful brochures about healthy bodies, coloring books, and stickers related to health and nursing. Demographic data, anecdotal records, parent and child verbal comments, and photographs were collected and analyzed. This initiative has had overwhelming success from the perspectives of the youth, parents, students, faculty, and community agencies involved.

Unintended and Concurrent Benefits: During the KIHC initiative, wellness and health promotion messages were also heard by young children. Parents attended events with children, and second careers in nursing were discussed. Discussions about nursing as a career crossed all age groups. Nursing students participated and learned age-appropriate health promotion and education skills. Requests from community agencies, schools, and senior centers to return were received consistently and continue to be received to the present day.

Because today's children will be tomorrow's health care providers, mechanisms to engage in this conversation in positive and fun ways are needed. Bringing nursing into the conscious thoughts of children, their parents, and other stakeholders may influence the future choice of a nursing career.

La Salle University School of Nursing and Health Sciences: "Kids into Health Careers"

La Salle University is located in an urban area in southeastern Pennsylvania. The "Kids into Health Careers" initiative implemented was supported by funding from the Division of Nursing (DN), Bureau of Health Professions (BHPr), Health Resources and Services Administration (HRSA), and the Department of Health and Human Services (DHHS). The "Kids into Health Careers" curriculum was developed based upon HRSA's existing curriculum, which focuses on informing participants that: 1) there are abundant job opportunities in health care; 2) qualifying for health care positions is rewarding; 3) financial aid is available; and 4) health care careers fill a critical need in many communities where minority and disadvantaged populations receive inadequate health care. During a two-year period, this initiative provided outreach and educational sessions at 26 public and private schools, targeting over 1,000 adolescents. A highlight of the KIHC initiative was a week-long summer camp event, conducted in July 2006, for participants from the school-based programs. Components of the camp included formal educational sessions, guest speakers who discussed their health careers, exposure to SIM man in the School of Nursing Learning Lab, and a mock disaster drill. Stethoscopes were provided to all participants and were used during the camp for hands-on learning. Reflective journaling revealed positive insights learned from this experience. This project was presented at the American Public Health Association Annual Meeting in Washington DC, November 5, 2007.

Other Types of Wellness Center Health Careers Initiatives

- Nurses can collaborate with the Girl and Boy Scouts, inviting them to the wellness center, where they can receive education about the services and care provided to clients. Nurses in the wellness center can have workshops that help the Scouts obtain their health-related badges.
- Wellness center staff can collaborate with guidance counselors of schools to coordinate day trips to the wellness center. Stations can be set up for students to provide hands-on learning. For example, students can learn how to listen to heart sounds, and take a pulse.
- Faculty can invite students to educational programs offered either at the wellness center or in an outreach setting, where nurses might arrange for willing clients to tell their stories of how a nurse made a difference in their lives.

▧ Wellness center directors can coordinate with faculty to incorporate service learning activity in their curriculum. A student or students could partner with a nurse from the wellness center to help with a teaching project or poster that can be posted in the center.

▧ Wellness Center staff can share the message that nursing is an intellectual profession that requires critical thinking. Messages can highlight that nurses make independent decisions within their scope of practice. Stories can be shared about how nurses make a difference in people's lives (Dunham & Smith, 2005; Sherrod, 2005).

▧ All involved in wellness center programmatic activities can share the video "Touching Lives, Changing Outcomes, A Tribute to Nurses," part of Johnson and Johnson's Campaign for Nursing's Future.

Conclusion

The KIHC initiative is one example of how nurses in wellness centers can partner with the community to result in added value to wellness centers by exposing young people to health care professional role models, which can influence children's lives and contribute positively to the future. This work is done locally through the wellness center's outreach activities but can have global impact. A caring and positive work environment in nursing wellness centers will contribute to the recruitment and retention of nurses wishing to do good work in ways that make a difference, particularly in the lives of the underserved.

Resources

http://www.aacn.nche.edu/media/shortageresource.htm
http://apha.confex.com/apha/135am/techprogram/paper_155327.htm
http://eric.ed.gov/ERICWebPortal/recordDetail?accno=ED463442
http://www.jbpub.com/catalog/9780763756840/
http://bhpr.hrsa.gov/KIDSCAREERS/about.htm
https://nursing.advanceweb.com/Editorial/Search/Aviewer.aspx?AN=NW06Jun12n1p16.html

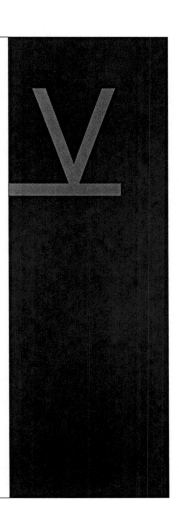

Improving and Measuring Quality in Wellness Centers

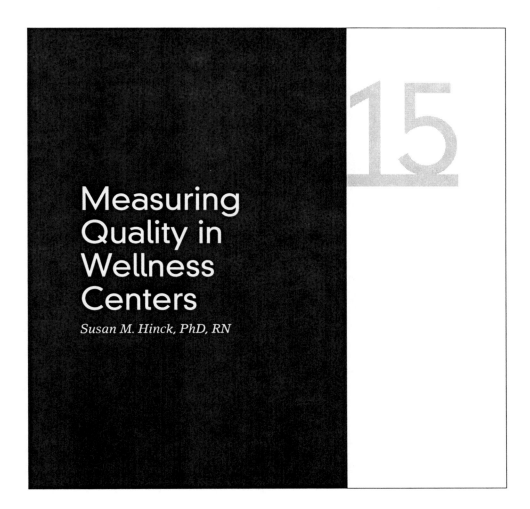

Measuring Quality in Wellness Centers

Susan M. Hinck, PhD, RN

Health Care Reform

The current health care system in the United States, which pays for the number of visits, tests and imaging, and procedures regardless of patient outcomes, pays most when treatment results in further injury or illness (IOM, 2001). In addition, the more than $2 trillion the U.S. spends each year for health care includes the cost of some care that is ineffective and not needed. Individuals receive evidence-based, recommended care less than 55% of the time (McGlynn et al., 2003). The cost of chronic illness care for very similar patients can cost more than twice as much in one area compared to other parts of the country. Increased costs are attributed to intensive use of resources, such as physician visits, medical specialist care (Baicker & Chandra, 2004), and advanced technology in diagnosis and treatment, without improvement in health outcomes. Unfortunately, more care does not mean better care. Patients who receive the most expensive treatments have worse outcomes, including higher mortality and less patient satisfaction, than those who receive more conservative care (Baicker & Chandra, 2004; Wennberg, Fisher, & Skinner, 2002).

Consumers and purchasers are demanding better value for their health care dollar. Public and private payers are electing to pay for quality of health care, instead of quantity of services. It is possible to have safe and effective care that meets the needs of individuals and populations, while at the same time reducing the cost of care (Berwick, Nolan, & Whittington, 2008; O'Kane et al., 2008). Payment tied to quality will reward providers for appropriate, effective, and efficient care.

According to the Institute of Medicine (IOM) *Crossing the Quality Chasm* report, quality care has the six components of safety, effectiveness (treatment that works), patient-centeredness, timeliness, efficiency (no overuse of unnecessary tests and treatment), and equity (IOM, 2001). Building on the Quality Chasm report, a series of three reports called *Pathways to Quality Health Care* were prepared by the IOM Committee on Redesigning Health Insurance Performance Measures, Payment, and Performance Improvement Programs. The titles of the three reports are *Medicare's Quality Improvement Organization Program: Maximizing Potential* (2006a), *Performance Measurement: Accelerating Improvement* (2006b), and *Rewarding Provider Performance: Aligning Incentives in Medicare* (2007). These reports promote a health system that contains the six components of quality care and is based on scientific evidence. All IOM reports can be viewed full-text online (www.nas.edu), although these are useful books to purchase and have in a professional library.

Wellness Care

As an alternative to pouring money into treating preventable diseases, prevention of disease through health education and health promotion is receiving increased attention. Wellness activities and programs are effective in preventing illnesses that can result in chronic disease, as well as in screening for disease at an early stage. Wellness centers provide health education, health promotion, and disease prevention services to individuals and families in communities. The need to learn to measure the quality and efficiency of care is important in nurse-managed wellness centers.

Past discussion of nursing center models has focused on delivery of care, with little attention to measurement of quality, cost, and the effectiveness of care (Murphy, 1995). However, provider accountability for care makes it necessary to know what interventions are effective for which individuals or groups, in order to provide high quality, efficient, and affordable health care. In a literature review, Coddington and Sands (2008) examined 10 studies reporting measures of quality and cost of primary care by advanced practice nurses in nurse-managed health clinics. Methods used to measure quality varied and included measures of patient satisfaction, quality of life, improvement in health, and functional status and independence. Investigators also reported that many nurse-managed clinics measured reductions in patient use of emergency departments and hospitalization. Few studies used national benchmarks in measuring quality. In some studies, costs were calculated per visit per patient, while other studies compared patient care cost at the clinic to other area primary care settings.

Measuring Quality

The five domains of health care quality measures are process, outcome, structure, resource use, and patient perception of experience. Processes are what the provider does. For example, a process measure of quality is whether an HgA1c was obtained for a diabetic patient. Outcome measures are what the patient does, with an example being whether the HgA1C reading was below 6. Structure measures are indirect measures of quality that have been empirically linked with a desired outcome. An example of a structure measure is the number and mix of nursing staff at the wellness center. Other examples of structure measures are the availability of an electronic decision support system for use by care providers, or electronic personal health records available for patients to view. Resource use is the cost of care over time for a patient or group of patients. Patient perception of experience is the use of a patient satisfaction survey to collect and report the consumer's input. Each domain can have multiple measures of quality.

Process measures are the most common measures used in quality improvement programs. In wellness centers, standardized process measurements of care identify whether research-based age- and sex-appropriate screening tests or interventions were offered. An example of a wellness outcome measure would be the measure of the proportion of the population practicing healthy lifestyle behaviors, such as tobacco cessation, increase in physical activity, or weight loss. Other recommendations for process measures for chronic care management are medication reconciliation across multiple primary care providers and education of patients about identification, purpose, and use of medications.

Public and private organizations have developed research-based measures of quality. Listings of measures that are nursing sensitive and related to wellness care can be found at Web sites of the Agency for Healthcare Research and Quality (AHRQ), Ambulatory Care Quality Alliance (ACQA), American Nurses Association (ANA), National Coalition of Quality (NCQA), and Institute of Medicine (IOM).

To support validity, a measure can undergo a systematic standardized process to be endorsed by a national organization. One such organization, the National Quality Forum (NQF), has been contracted by the Centers for Medicare and Medicaid Services (CMS) to endorse measures used in federal pay-for-performance programs. NQF is a private, nonprofit, open membership, public benefit corporation, established in 1999. The endorsement process begins with a call for nomination of measures. Measures can be nominated by individuals, professional organizations, clinical groups, or academics. NQF staff and the Consensus Standard Approval Committee (CSAC) evaluate the measures and then the measures are electronically posted for public comment. The evaluation is based on the importance (need for improvement), scientific acceptability (level of evidence to support the measure), usability (used in clinical settings), and feasibility (implementation with little burden) of the measure. The more than 300 NQF organization members vote on endorsement. The CSAC and the NQF Board of Directors give final approval. Measures then have an appeal period before final endorsement. NQF has endorsed 15 nursing care-sensitive process, structure, and outcome measures, as well as hundreds of measures for care in various settings.

Over the past 15 years, the American Nurses Association has developed a National Database of Nursing Quality Indicators (NDNQI) for reporting structure, process, and outcome indicators for hospital units (Montalvo, 2007). To provide a comprehensive overview of measures of nursing quality, Rantz, Bostick, and Riggs (2002) conducted a literature review of over 300 research articles that measured quality care in hospital, nursing home, home health, community health, and ambulatory care settings. Existing quality indicators may be revised where needed and adopted for use in measuring quality of health promotion programs in wellness centers. For example, the recommendation of immunizations for hospitalized patients may be a relevant quality indicator for patients in non-hospital settings.

Physicians take part in measuring and public reporting of quality indicators of ambulatory care. The 2006 Tax Relief and Health Care Act mandated the use of the Physician Quality Reporting Initiative (PQRI) system for Medicare providers. Physicians voluntarily reported process and outcome quality indicators from July 1 to December 31, 2007, and received a bonus payment, subject to a cap, equal to 1.5% of their total allowed Medicare charges for the six-month period. The PQRI program continues and will change from paying for reporting to paying for meeting benchmarks, and will eventually become mandatory.

Bundling Measures

Measures can be grouped into episodes of illness so that provider efficiency can be measured and reported by illness (http//:www.medPAC.gov/documents/Jun06_EntireReport.pdf). For example, the Diabetes Quality Improvement Project to measure quality of care for diabetic patients has been a joint venture involving providers, specialty organizations, and quality assurance organizations (IOM, 2001). Some samples of quality measures bundled for Diabetes Mellitus are the 10 actions listed in Table 15.1.

15.1 Ten Actions for Diabetes Mellitus	
DM-1 HbA1c Management	DM-6 Urine Protein Testing
DM-2 HbA1c Control	DM-7 Eye Exam
DM-3 Blood Pressure Management	DM-8 Foot Exam
DM-4 Lipid Measurement	DM-9 Influenza Vaccination
DM-5 LDL Cholesterol Level	DM-10 Pneumonia Vaccination

Transparency of Quality and Cost

Public reporting of aggregate measurement data is a powerful vehicle to drive quality improvement (IOM, Pathways to Quality Health Care Series, 2006 & 2007). The Centers for Medicare and Medicaid Services publically report quality measures for hospitals and will soon post quality measures for other settings of care, including ambulatory care, home health, hospice, and nursing home settings. So far, quality measures of hospital care for patients who have been admitted with heart attack, heart failure, or pneumonia diagnoses or patients having surgery are available on Hospital Compare at the CMS Quality of Care Center accessible at www.cms.gov. Comparison can be made for facilities in a specific zip code or by facility name. Additional quality measures will be posted on the site as they are added.

Barriers to Implementing Quality Measures

Barriers to implementing quality measures are the cost in time, dollars, and training for data collection and management. The lack of a standard electronic health record (EHR) to automate the process of gathering, analyzing, storing, and distributing unit-level data often prevents comprehensive measurement. A fully integrated EHR and decision support system embeds the data elements and produces the nursing measures as a byproduct of care. Software containing the measures should be in one integrated EHR system to meet the needs of the payer (billing), regulator, consumer (viewable personal health record), and any accreditor (Corrigan, 2007). Fully integrated EHRs are rare, with the exception of the Veterans' Administration's closed system and the Kaiser Permanente system. Most facilities use multiple software systems with billing separate from the electronic patient record, and the system often cannot communicate with outside systems.

Payment for Wellness Services

Often, payment for wellness care is incorporated into primary care and is not singled out as a separate payment code. This has been a financial dilemma for nurse-managed wellness centers and primary care providers that emphasize health education and illness prevention. Payment for quality care, instead of payment based on the quantity of services provided and billed, has been a recent focus of CMS. Pay-for-performance, called a Value-Based Purchasing (VBP) program by CMS, financially rewards or penalizes providers according to performance on select quality measures. VBP applies to a small share of the clinician's fee-for-service Medicare revenue. The VBP plan can be used to improve quality of care in all settings, including hospital, physician, nursing home, hospice, and home health services (IOM, Pathways to Quality Health Care Series, 2006 & 2007).

Conclusion

Quality care improves patient outcomes and lowers cost. Measures of quality in nurse-managed wellness centers should be nationally standardized and publically reported so that potential patients can make informed decisions about their choice of providers, clinicians in wellness centers can view their own performance in relation to centers across the country, and quality and cost comparisons can be made across geographic areas.

Resources

Agency for Healthcare Research and Quality (AHRQ). www.ahrq.gov
Ambulatory Care Quality Alliance (ACQA). www.ambulatoryqualityalliance.org
American Nurses Association (ANA). www.nursingworld.org
Centers for Medicare and Medicaid Services (CMS) Quality of Care Center. www.cms.gov
Dartmouth Atlas of Health Care. www.dartmouthatlas.org
Institute of Medicine, National Academies of Science (IOM). www.nas.edu
Medicare Payment Advisory Commission. www.medpac.gov
National Coalition of Quality (NCQA). www.ncqa.org
National Quality Forum. www.qualityforum.org

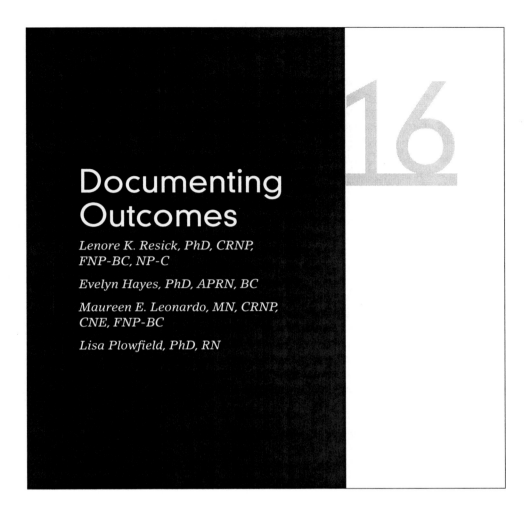

Documenting Outcomes

Lenore K. Resick, PhD, CRNP, FNP-BC, NP-C

Evelyn Hayes, PhD, APRN, BC

Maureen E. Leonardo, MN, CRNP, CNE, FNP-BC

Lisa Plowfield, PhD, RN

Introduction

This chapter discusses the common challenges encountered when documenting wellness center outcomes. Commonly used documentation systems are presented along with a discussion of the experiences of two wellness centers. This chapter ends with lists and examples of some helpful documentation resources.

Commonly Encountered Challenges Regarding Documentation

Although quantifying outcomes of health promotion and wellness interventions is essential to ongoing operations of nurse-managed wellness centers, documentation of outcomes related to health promotion and wellness interventions present many challenges. Traditional documentation systems are based on a medical model and disease paradigm. These systems are designed for use in short-term, acute care and traditional medical model primary care settings. Unlike outcome measures based on a disease paradigm, wellness outcome measurements may not be defined points after interventions, since wellness is a long-term objective not easily linked to single care events. For example, in a wellness setting focused on the care of older adults, the desired outcome may not be a change in status or improvement, but stabilization of the patient's health status.

Outcomes defined and measured in a traditional primary care model nursing center may not be applicable to those outcomes defined and measured in a wellness model of care center. Documentation and coding systems such as the *Current Procedural Terminology* (CPT) (American Medical Association, 2008), which is the standard used for billing in traditional primary care models of nursing centers, often do not capture the essence of environmental and social problems and other variables that contribute to outcomes related to wellness interventions.

Renewable grant funding and ongoing operation of wellness centers require documented "outcomes." These outcomes require the collection of data related to client wellness as a result of nursing interventions. Outcomes also involve outcomes related to the satisfaction of clients using the services of the wellness centers, in addition to the satisfaction of wellness center staff and the community in which the wellness center is located. For academic wellness centers, outcomes include faculty scholarship, faculty and student satisfaction, and student learning outcomes. More broadly defined, outcomes are also directly related to the needs assessment, goals, and objectives of the wellness center.

Determining the Purpose and Goals of Documentation

The collection of outcome data occurs in many ways. Some essential questions to consider in preparing to collect data include the following: Why are data needed?, What data need to be collected to give the information needed?, How are data to be collected, recorded, and stored for accessibility? (Wade, 2004). The data collection tool to be used is an important consideration. Wade identifies the following questions to ask when choosing any data collection tool: Will this data collection tool:

- Collect the data needed to answer my question? (Is it valid for my purpose?)
- Give the level of certainty required? (Is it sufficiently reliable?)
- Detect the extent of change or difference expected? (Is it adequately sensitive?)
- Be practical in the circumstances? (Can it and will it be used?)
- Give information that can be understood by those needing information? (Can the results be communicated easily?) (Wade, 2004, p. 235)

Challenges of Commonly Used Formats for Documenting Care in Wellness Centers

Several formats exist for documenting care in wellness centers. These include Nursing Interventions Classification (NIC) (Dochterman & Bulechek, 2004), Nursing Outcomes Classification (NOC) (Moorhead, Johnson, & Maas, 2004), and the Omaha System (Martin & Scheet, 1992). These commonly used documenta-tion systems offer some very useful aspects for documentation needs in wellness centers. For example, the NIC, which is a list of nursing interventions developed by the Iowa Intervention Project, has been used successfully by parish nurses working with client aggregates with a focus on health promotion and disease prevention in the community (Weiss, Schank, Coenen, & Matheus, 2002). The Omaha System is multifunctional and provides the ability to document wellness activities and care, education, and surveillance in acute, chronic, and primary care. In addition, the Omaha System permits documentation to reflect individual clients, families, communities, and populations. These documentation systems do not use a common language and intercoder reliability is often difficult to achieve between two care providers using the same system in the same nursing center.

Experiences From Two Wellness Centers: Lessons Learned

University of Delaware (UD) Nursing Center

Although documentation of outcomes can be both qualitative and quantitative, Martin and Scheet (1992) indicate that client record data too often end up bur-ied in the "data cemetery," not a desired result. Meaningful data management requires special skills and planning from inception (actually, in pre-inception) of a project. The data collected with the Omaha System can be meaningful and reliably used to address clients' needs and services to meet these needs.

Prevention services and outcomes can be examined by analyzing documen-tation for problems assessed as potential or health promotion. Knowing the impact of a program on a target population is highly desirable and expected in many situations. The Sure Start Program in Wales is an example of a suc-cessful program, where the "Knowledge-Behavior-Status" ratings were used to document the program's effectiveness and helped to secure ongoing funding (Christiansen, Koudos, & Clark, 2005).

Data management is crucial to the successful evaluation of the outcomes of any project. The experience at UD with data collection was challenging and provided a number of "lessons learned." User-friendly surveys were used that had multiple data points to be collected. Missing data and unusable data in one section on the survey and some miscommunication with community resources signaled a definite need for a more rigorous orientation of both faculty and students to the survey tool and its use. It is essential that all users of the sur-vey understand not only the individual components, but also the interrelation-ship/triggering effect impairment can have on further description. Vigilance is required throughout the process of data collection to be certain that students conducting the surveys understand them fully and that all appropriate data are addressed and recorded with each client encounter. Student and faculty review of the data for completeness and accuracy needs to be done on a daily basis.

The UD Nursing Center adapted the Omaha System for documentation related to the Comprehensive Geriatric Assessment (CGA). Modifications included organizing the data in a head-to-toe format consistent with an interdisciplinary standard/format. A second modification was the addition of two areas, including the breast health and examination and the "Head, Eyes, Ears, Nose and Throat (HEENT)" section. Please refer to Appendix D-18 for the complete assessment tool.

Data from the Omaha System has been the foundation of an aspect of the scholarship of the UD Nursing Center team. Examples of this scholarship follow:

- Using the Omaha System to collect and analyze the comprehensive needs of community-dwelling elders led to the identification of residential safety hazards. A case study analysis and retrospective chart review approach were used to examine the meaning of clutter for those frail elders who exhibited this environmental need. Analysis of nine Omaha System needs was conducted using a CGA record review. The needs included: residence, income, health care supervision, communication with community resources, caretaking, cognition, nutrition, interpersonal relationships, and social contact. Trends were identified for further study. Another study based on the Omaha System of documentation is "Exploring Issues of Social Isolation in Frail Elderly." Based on current definitions of social isolation, two psychosocial needs, interpersonal relationships, and social contact were selected to study this phenomenon. Data were compared from the 1996–2001 cohort with the 2005–2006 cohort.
- Use of the Omaha System for documentation with targeted surveys was also designed as part of the Promoting Healthy Lifestyles in Delaware Project. Targeted surveys include: Blood Pressure/Stroke Risk Screening, Nutrition, and General Health Inventory. In addition, a one page Omaha System Information Sheet was developed. Please refer to Appendix D-18.

Duquesne University School of Nursing Nurse-Managed Wellness Center

Since 1994, the Duquesne University School of Nursing Nurse-Managed Wellness Center (DUSON NMWC) has provided on-site health promotion and wellness services to older adults residing in two older adult high-rise apartment buildings. Through a collaborative agreement with the City of Pittsburgh Department of Parks and Recreation, DUSON NMWC services now include health and wellness services to community-dwelling older adults who attend community senior centers in ten additional ethnically diverse Pittsburgh neighborhoods. These wellness sites are staffed by volunteer registered nurses, nursing faculty who are advanced practice nurses, and undergraduate and graduate nursing students.

Three categories of outcomes are evaluated: 1) nursing student-centered outcomes that include student satisfaction, learning, and faculty satisfaction, 2) program outcomes that include numbers of participating clients, client satisfaction, and changes in clients' health-related behaviors, and 3) client-centered outcomes measured by management of chronic disease, identification and management of health risks, and delay of functional decline (Taylor, Resick, D'Antonio, & Carroll, 1997).

The clients of the DUSON NMWC typically live independently and remain active, and their chronic medical conditions are relatively stable. However, they are also aging in place and, due to advanced aging and progression of chronic disease conditions, are experiencing decreasing function. Consistently, needs assessments of this population have indicated the need for health and wellness services.

Documenting outcomes of care of older adults in a community wellness center presents many challenges. Typically, interactions are brief and sporadic and clients may have a wide range of health and wellness needs. Accurate assessment of baseline data involving recall by older adults is a particular challenge, so this assessment data may need to be validated. The majority of client visits focus on problems with circulation and nutrition. The most common intervention categories continue to be Health Teaching, Guidance, Counseling, and Surveillance.

During the early evolution of the Duquesne University Nurse Managed Wellness Center, the Omaha System was adapted to categorize the reason for encounters and Focus Charting® (Lampe, 1997) was used to organize anecdotal notes (Resick, Taylor, & Leonardo, 1999). Since documentation was done manually using this combined system of Omaha and Focus Charting® (Lampe, 1997), tracking outcomes over time for trends involved thematic analysis. Abstracting data consistently and accurately was a challenge. As a result, a large quantity of data was lost in the narratives, and thematic analysis was not an efficient or reasonable method to quantify outcomes, and data analysis resulted in the discovery of inconsistencies in documentation. This finding suggested that, although the Omaha System has provided a useful and reliable framework for generating reliable data, data collection, and analysis, an ongoing process for learning and validating intercoder reliability was essential to maintaining rigor of data collection within and among the various wellness center sites (Leonardo, Resick, Bingman, & Strotmeyer, 2004).

It was clear that a computerized system of documentation was essential for adequate data analysis. After initially working manually with the combination of the Omaha System and Focus Charting® (Lampe, 1997) documentation systems, the staff realized the need to move data into an electronic format for ease in record keeping and meaningful data analysis. The decision was made to move totally toward using the Omaha System alone for documentation. In addition, various additional forms were developed to track blood pressure readings, weights, medications, and health maintenance schedules.

Staff found that, although using a laptop computer to record data directly onto a form during client encounters is time efficient, this created a barrier between client and nurse. As a result, client information is documented during the encounter using paper and pen and later entered into the automated system. SPSS Data Builder (Norusis, 2002) was used to create customized data entry forms and perform data entry functions. This structure permitted categorical and continuous data to be collected to form a longitudinal database. Each client is assigned a 5-digit code and computer access is limited to those directly involved in care or data entry and analysis.

Finally, data analysis did not capture the outcomes related to human experiences. For example, measurements of program ownership and the experience of health and wellness are difficult outcomes to measure. Currently, the nurses are working toward developing a qualitative aspect to data collection to better interpret the human experiences of health and wellness. The ultimate goal is to provide services that facilitate self-care, a high level of wellness, and improvement in the quality of life.

Last Notes

The following section includes a summary of questions to consider when choosing a documentation system and a data management system for a wellness center.

Questions to consider when choosing a documentation system:

- Is the documentation system interdisciplinary and research based?
- Is the system user-friendly and student-friendly?
- What are the research capabilities for outcomes documentation?
- Is the documentation system based on a standardized language and recognized as one of 13 accepted standardized documentation systems?
- Does the system provide adequate automated/technical capabilities?
- To what extent is the documentation practical to use in a wellness model of care? (Consider targeted surveys versus comprehensive needs analyses)
- What is the ease of monitoring intercoder reliability or universal understanding of the system and coding?

Questions to consider when choosing a data management system:

- Will paper tools be used or will data be entered directly into a computer?
- What confidentiality checks are in place?
- What are the data entry requirements?
- How will data be checked to determine correct entry? (Is there a quality assurance process in place that includes an evaluation process for correction of errors?)
- How data will be analyzed and used?
- How aggregate data will be managed?

Resources

http://www.omahasystem.org/
http://www.omahasystem.org/referenc.htm
http://www.omahasystem.org/links.htm
http://www.nanda.org/index.html
The Web site for the University of Iowa College of Nursing Center for Nursing Classification & Clinical Effectiveness: http://www.nursing.uiowa.edu/excellence/nursingknowledge/clinicaleffectiveness/index.htm.

17

Data Collection

Eunice S. King, PhD, RN

M. Elaine Tagliareni, EdD, RN

Nurses have historically played a critical role in the delivery of community-based health promotion programs and services essential to achieving the Healthy People Objectives for the Nation (U.S. Department of Health and Human Services, 2000). In wellness centers, nurses focus primarily on providing community-based health promotion programs and services to diverse populations. Some of these services occur in individual sessions between the client and the nurse, whereas others are offered in group settings. In all instances, however, the nature of the services and the delivery mode are determined by a needs assessment regarding the target populations served and through unique and productive relationships with community partners and residents.

In spite of the importance of these programs in promoting the health of the communities and constituencies served, funding to support them has been problematic and has come largely from foundations and highly competitive governmental grants. As funding for such programs has become increasingly scarce, the availability of supporting data that document program outcomes and/or service needs has become imperative. These data can strengthen grant applications, are important when submitting reports to funders, and can often help identify additional existing and future target population needs.

Although many publicly funded health promotion programs, such as Lead Safe Babies and Asthma Safe Kids, disseminated through the National Nursing Centers Consortium (NNCC, 2005), or Lead Awareness North Philly Style (Rothman, Lourie, & Gaughan, 2002), have data collection criteria built in as critical components of program evaluation, most centers offer many services and programs that do not include formal evaluation processes. Consequently, systems for collecting data that document the scope of services provided and clients served have been disparate, often limited to paper and pencil tabulations, and sometimes sporadic at best. The need for an electronic system for the collection of health promotion program data was identified as early as the mid-1990s by several Independence Foundation grantee applicants, later by a number of HRSA, Division of Nursing grantees (Anderko & Kinion, 2001), and most recently by networks of nurse practitioners under grants from the Agency for Healthcare Research and Quality (AHRQ) (Deshefy-Longhi, Swartz, & Grey, 2008). Although electronic data collection systems are being utilized in many nurse-managed wellness centers, most have been designed to collect primary care and practice management-related data and often require extensive programming modifications to capture health promotion data. Furthermore, even when they can be modified, capturing health promotion data on clients who are not also primary care clients can be very problematic. Thus, nurse-managed centers offering exclusively wellness services have had very limited options for an electronic data collection tool.

Challenges in Collecting Health Promotion Data

Collection of data describing participants in health promotion programs can be very challenging for many reasons. Many attendees of group programs dislike completing forms, even brief surveys that collect basic demographic data. Some are unable to complete the forms without personal assistance, which might not be available, and, in some situations, dread of surveys and forms can be a deterrent to program attendance. Older adults in particular do not like to complete paper and pencil surveys, often due to visual impairments and writing difficulties imposed by arthritis, tremors, etc. Some facilities where health promotion programs are conducted, such as schools and congregate living facilities, have strict policies that preclude outside agencies from collecting data regarding students' or residents' personal information. Often, public health decision-making is evidence-based and depends on high quality and transparent accounts of what interventions are effective, for whom, how, and at what cost to the center and to the resident. Yet, collection of data describing the impact of health promotion programs can be difficult and often requires use of individual baseline patient encounter information to determine change and impact of programming. Consequently, program outcome data are most often described in the aggregate and information regarding the overall impact of the intervention may be limited.

Prior to developing or adopting a tool, it is essential that a center carefully assess the nature of its existing programs as well as the data reporting requirements of program funders and attempt to anticipate future data needs. In addition, it should create a list of questions about the services it provides and insure that the data collection tool will capture the data needed.

Community College of Philadelphia Health Promotion Data Collection Tool

In December 2000, the Independence Foundation awarded a grant to the Community College of Philadelphia (CCP) to support the development and testing of an electronic data collection tool to describe and document the scope of common health promotion/disease prevention activities. To circumvent the problems commonly encountered in collecting health promotion data, the CCP instrument was designed to collect data anonymously and to be completed by one of the professional or nursing student program providers in a minimal amount of time, so as not to detract from service delivery, yet still allow for the capture of important data about the scope of services provided and characteristics of the clients served. The data were to be used to describe client characteristics, as well as the number and scope of services provided. Periodic reports documenting the number and type of health promotion/disease prevention services and programs offered, the number of clients served, and their characteristics, could be generated for each of the participating centers and for the NNCC. Once the tool had undergone testing and revisions by the pilot centers, it was anticipated that it would ultimately be available for use by additional NNCC member centers.

During the first year of tool development, CCP faculty, under the leadership of Dr. Elaine Tagliareni, worked with students to develop a paper and pencil form that was completed after each health promotion activity conducted as part of students' clinical practica in the 19130 Zip Code Project, a wellness center without walls, and then entered in a computer database. After multiple revisions to the paper instrument and consultation with CCP's information technology department, the form was converted to an electronic one accessed through the Internet. It became clear after the first year, that two slightly different versions of the data collection tool would be needed: one for health promotion activities conducted in groups, such as exercise classes or health education programs, and the other for those conducted in individual settings, such as individual counseling or brown bag medication reviews. All referrals made following or during group encounters were considered to be "individual data."

Since it was important to validate tool utility and fit for centers providing disparate services and targeting a wide range of clients, the tool was tested in seven NNCC-affiliated nursing centers that served divergent populations in rural, urban, and suburban settings. Four of those centers offered exclusively wellness services and three provided both primary care and wellness services. Each offered a wide range of health promotion services and programs based upon: a) a needs assessment of the local community, in collaboration with strategic key informants, and b) guidelines specified in the Healthy People 2010 Goals for the Nation (USDHHS, 2000) for the specific target populations served. In some centers, the needs assessment dictated programming toward specific target groups (e.g., teaching about immunizations to parents of toddlers and pre-schoolers participating in Head Start Programs; conducting medication "brown bag" events in senior high-rise apartment complexes) and toward meeting outcomes established through local funding initiatives (e.g., development of a lead screening and awareness program in response to increased lead levels in an urban environment; establishment of a cardiovascular health promotion program for high-risk adults in a rural community where access to primary care providers was limited).

Healthy People 2010 objectives, specifically those related to educational and community-based programs, provided benchmarks for targeting specific programming to improve access to information about prevention of suicide and depression, tobacco use, HIV/AIDS, STD infection, unhealthy dietary patterns, cardiovascular health, and cancer awareness. All other initiatives were directed towards achieving the Healthy People 2010 goals of increasing the proportion of residents from high-risk populations (e.g., pre-school children and parents, middle, junior and senior high school students, adults over age 65) who receive consistent and supportive health care information. Over the next four to five years, the participating pilot centers met annually to assess the instrument's ability to adequately capture important data, to identify problems impacting its ease and accuracy, and to recommend revisions.

Tool Description

The CCP Health Promotion Data Collection Tool organizes health promotion activities into one of two categories, both of which are based on selected nursing intervention categories specified by the Omaha System (Martin, Leak, & Aden, 1997):

■ *Health Teaching, Guidance, and Counseling*: Included within this category is health teaching on topics that include dental care, safety, cardiovascular care, human growth and development, nutrition, medication action and side effects, lead poisoning prevention, and exercise, to name a few. Anticipating client problems, encouraging client action and responsibility for self-care and coping, and assisting with decision making and problem solving related to managing one's health and life are guidance and counseling activities also included in this category. "Advocacy for health and life management" is also included in this category, in order to adequately capture the scope of services most often provided to clients aged 65 and older, e.g., helping the client arrange transportation, calling pharmacies on behalf of patients, and negotiating reimbursement with insurance carriers. For those centers that targeted wellness services directly to older adults, finding a way to capture the center's advocacy role is crucial.

■ *Surveillance, Detection, Measurement, Critical Analysis, and/or Monitoring Clients' Status in Relation to a Given Condition or Phenomenon*: Examples of these activities are height and weight measurement, vision and hearing screening, glucose monitoring, blood pressure evaluation, and scoliosis screening. Clients with abnormal findings are referred to other agencies or providers for services and followed by the wellness center staff. For each category, a list of activities, specific enough to be informative, yet generic enough to capture all centers' activities, was developed and modified multiple times over the course of the tool's development. A "data dictionary," with explicit directions and examples of how activities should be coded was developed and underwent extensive testing and revision.

Procedures for Tool Use

During each group session, a designated recorder counts the number of participants and categorizes them according to racial background and broad age groups,
e.g., 20 attendees, all aged 60 or older, 10 African American, 5 White, and 5 Asian.
Demographic and health care utilization data collected for individual encounters
are self-reported through interviews with clients. For children seen in Head Start
programs or in elementary schools, agency records are utilized. If data are not
available, they are recorded as unknown.

Data collected during group-directed activities or encounters are referred
to as "group data" and reflect total attendance at all programs. Each program
attendee is considered an encounter. Because many individuals attended
more than one program, the total number of encounters is a duplicated count,
reflecting total attendance at programs, not the total of individual participants.
"Individual data" refer to sessions between the nurse and a client in a nursing center, a community agency, school, or the client's home and often occur
subsequent to a group encounter. For example, all participants with abnormal
screening results are referred to the appropriate provider and the individual
encounter tool is completed to record the type of referral made. As with the
"group data," the aggregate number of individual encounters could include
multiple sessions with the same client and thus do not reflect the number of
individual clients served.

After recording client characteristics, the nurse checks all services provided
during the course of the session, regardless of type (group or individual). For
example, a health education class on managing cardiovascular disease could
include information about signs and symptoms of cardiovascular disease, medication action and side effects, and nutrition counseling. These data are then
entered into the electronic database accessed on the Internet.

Benefits and Limitations of the Tool

The process and data collected over the four-year period of development of the
Health Promotion Data Collection Tool have guided numerous revisions to the
instrument, which has now been effectively tested and utilized in seven wellness nursing centers. The tool has been found to adequately capture the scope
of activities and services provided and to accurately characterize the clients
served. When the data have been examined by individual centers, there has
emerged considerable variation reflective of the unique demographic characteristics of the communities served. This has led to the understanding that
wellness centers are not homogeneous, and that services provided are dictated
by the needs and characteristics of the community and populations served. For
example, one wellness center has local funding to provide a wide range of services to address the incidence of lead poisoning in the area; therefore aggregate data from this center showed a large percentage of services related to lead
awareness teaching, screening for developmental milestones, and health advocacy. In another center where the population served is older adults who live in a
senior high rise building, data revealed a high percentage of nutrition teaching,
as well as cardiovascular screening and medication management.

Due to the collaborative efforts of project staff and representatives from all seven centers, the Health Promotion Data Collection Tool that was developed can potentially be used by any wellness nursing center to capture the range of services provided and characteristics of clients served. Furthermore, while the pilot centers originally sought to develop a tool that addressed the unique characteristics of their centers and regions, what emerged was a generic tool that has yielded data reflective of the comprehensive nature of the services provided and the clients served, without becoming so specific that it is difficult to use. Hence, it has been well accepted and used by staff in the participating centers to document their work.

Very importantly, the data collected have been used to generate additional questions to be addressed. For example, after the first year of use by all seven pilot centers, a report was generated for each individual center as well as one showing the aggregate data (Tagliareni & King, 2006). In examining the patterns of usage and services across centers, it became clear that a major group of consumers of health promotion activities, both individual and group directed, were adults aged 60 and older and that the services provided in fact were those that augment those of primary care providers and may contribute to seniors' ability to maintain independent living. During a six-month reporting period, the health and life management category, which included helping clients arrange transportation, calling pharmacies on behalf of patients, assisting with contacting insurance carriers, and conducting group programs on topics such as "How to Use Your Medicare Prescription Benefit," comprised a fifth of the individual encounters with clients aged 60 and older. These services, as well as many others, offered to clients in senior citizens' housing communities, were potentially facilitating independent living and clients' management of complex chronic health problems. In addition, many of the health teaching topics offered to older adults during the same period, e.g., education on medication action/side effects, cardiovascular education, hypertension management, and diabetic care education, also potentially helped them maintain their independence. This data led to additional questions about the importance of nursing centers' role in enabling older adults manage their health issues and sustain functional independence. The questions raised have spawned an in-depth pilot, qualitative study to explore how nurse-managed wellness centers assist senior adults in maintaining independent living.

Although this data collection tool has enabled the centers using it to adequately document the scope of services provided, to describe their clients, and to identify questions for further study, it is not without its limitations. It does not accommodate descriptions of program specificity. Furthermore, the descriptions of client characteristics, particularly of clients attending group programs, are obtained from observers and subject to error. Finally, questions about service utilization by individuals cannot be addressed because the data are entered into the system anonymously.

The most important limitation of this tool is its inability to capture health outcome data. That is because the instrument was envisioned to be used in situations where collection of data that could be linked to discrete individuals was often problematic. Hence, tracking of specific individuals' use of services and changes in health status is not possible and the impact of these services and programs on actual health outcomes cannot be evaluated.

Recommendations

Prior to adopting an existing data collection tool, it is extremely important that a center first assess its own data collection needs. The following questions can be a helpful guide in the assessment process:

- What do we or our funders want to know about the services provided and the clients served?
- What data do we want to collect? Descriptive or outcome data?
- What are the challenges anticipated in collecting those data?
- How will we generate reports from the data set?
- What do we anticipate our future data needs will be?
- How much will the data collection tool/system cost, both for the initial purchase or development and for ongoing maintenance?

Conclusions

In addition to the data collection tool detailed here, there are several others being utilized to document health promotion services (Lundeen, 1999). The consistent data elements in the tools are the types and patterns of services provided and constituencies served across the life span. During the time that these descriptive tools have been utilized by wellness centers, considerable revisions have been accomplished and they have been found to be reliable instruments. However, documenting the scope of services provided and describing the program participants is not sufficient for demonstrating the value of nurse-managed wellness centers to promoting the health of communities. There is a need now to systematically collect data related to program outcomes and program effectiveness, thereby documenting impact of health promotion programs, targeted at specific populations. It is only through the documentation of program outcomes that wellness centers will capture the attention of health policy makers and demonstrate the value of their work.

Appendices

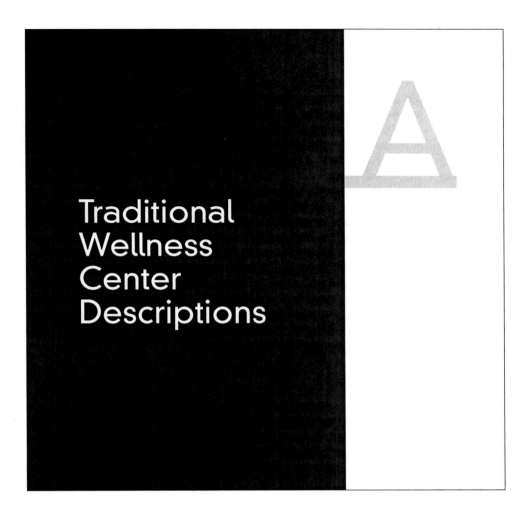

Traditional Wellness Center Descriptions

Coalition for Healthy Communities, Springfield, Missouri

Development of a Wellness Center Without Walls

Springfield, Missouri, is a community in a large, metropolitan area that is characterized by urban and rural populations that are homeless and uninsured and have low health-literacy levels. Service organizations meet some needs of this population, but access to health care is restricted. Nursing programs at Missouri State University (MSU) have a long history of providing community-based nursing education to undergraduate and graduate students. The university's philosophy of community-based nursing education programs is to work collaboratively to meet the learning needs of the students, the service needs of the agency, and the health needs of the population served. The Coalition for Healthy Communities (CHC) started with a vision to engage undergraduate BSN generic and completion nursing students in service-learning activities to deliver basic, population-focused nursing care to vulnerable populations that did not have access to nurses.

Establishment of a "wellness center without walls" was envisioned to enable nursing students to meet population health needs at different locations within the community. The center was designed to provide a structure for student clinical experiences in the nursing program, as well as to provide a rich environment for student and faculty research. Placing a number of students in close proximity in a limited number of areas utilized the clinical supervisor's time effectively.

The nursing wellness center without walls began in the spring semester of 2005 with one partner organization to serve high-risk mothers and families. Coalition for Healthy Communities now has two partner organizations with seven sites and serves individuals, families, and groups, composed of a diverse range of ages (infancy through old age) and ethnic backgrounds. One common thread among all nursing center sites is that the populations are vulnerable, experiencing acute or chronic poverty, uninsured, and in crisis. Two nursing professors, working with nursing students, developed and implemented CHC. The center is based on four theoretical perspectives: (1) service-learning approach, (2) student-to-student peer mentoring, (3) Patricia Benner's Novice to Expert Model (Benner, 1984), and (4) community- and evidence-based nursing practice.

Mission Statement

The mission of CHC is to promote the health and well-being of at-risk individuals, families, and groups by providing essential community health care through collaboration between Missouri State University (MSU) Department of Nursing and contracted agencies. Coalition for Healthy Communities strives to facilitate care through education to empower individuals and improve health outcomes of the community served.

The philosophy of CHC is based on the idea that human beings are unique due to diverse genetic endowments and personal experiences in social and physical environments, and on the idea that humans have the ability to adapt to biophysical, psychosocial, and spiritual stressors. Therefore, each person is considered a unique individual with unique needs.

Services

Coalition for Healthy Communities supports individuals, families, and groups in setting priorities, identifying goals and outcomes, and striving for mutual trust and understanding. The MSU student nurse collaborates with the contracted agency to increase individuals' and families' knowledge base about health. Services provided by students participating in CHC are grouped into two categories of leadership/management and community health activities:

1. Leadership and management activities, which include:
   - Development and update of current mission, philosophy, purpose, goals, strategic plan, organizational chart, and policies and procedures
   - Staff education and training, covering such topics as blood-borne pathogens precaution, interdisciplinary assessment procedure, and how to assist a client having a seizure

2. Community health assessment, education, and referral activities performed by students, which include:
   - Assessing individuals, families, groups, and communities
   - Developing and implementing health fairs and screening
   - Providing information that is culturally competent and health-literacy appropriate
   - Providing health-promotion and disease-management information
   - Clarifying prescription medication information
   - Referring individuals, families, or groups to accessible and affordable health providers

Performing procedures is a minor role fulfilled by students at the center. Examples include the administration of flu vaccine and assisting individuals with basic nursing care, such as wound care.

Outcomes are measured by collection of data following assessment, educational sessions, and referral. To ensure client satisfaction, clients are verbally questioned about their care. A specific tool for client or agency satisfaction with the wellness center has not been implemented at this time.

Staffing

Two full-time nursing faculty who teach community health as well as leadership and management courses oversee CHC and serve as liaisons with the community agencies. One 32-hour-per-week clinical supervisor is assigned to CHC to facilitate learning and to evaluate undergraduate nursing students. The faculty and supervisor salaries are paid through the MSU Department of Nursing budget. The nursing students are placed in roles to lead and manage the wellness clinic, and to implement the nursing roles of assessment, education, and referral. Each student who is assigned to the center is enrolled in a service-learning course and spends 64–96 hours at the Center. The number of undergraduate nursing students assigned to the CHC ranges from 30 to 45 per semester. Each of the wellness center sites is open for 8 hours (specific hours vary by location) on Tuesdays and Thursdays during the academic fall and spring semesters because students are available at that time. Nursing faculty supervise and are available to nursing students at all times.

Population Served

Coalition for Healthy Communities serves vulnerable individuals, families, and groups at seven sites. Most individuals evaluated at the wellness centers are experiencing homelessness or are poverty stricken, uninsured, and in a state of acute or chronic crisis. Health and social conditions frequently seen are mental illnesses, substance abuse, violence, neglect, trauma, hyperthermia, hypothermia, hypertension, diabetes, and a variety of acute and chronic lung diseases. The population is culturally diverse, with these ethnic groups being served: Caucasian, African American, Native American, Hispanic, and Asian. All are experiencing the culture of poverty.

Reimbursement

Coalition for Healthy Communities is supported by the MSU Department of Nursing and the collaborating agencies: The Kitchen and Victory Mission. The MSU Department of Nursing provides faculty to coordinate and supervise nursing student service-learning experiences at the seven wellness center sites for up to four days a week during the fall and spring academic semesters. The Kitchen and Victory Mission provide the space, supplies, and technology for the wellness clinic. Both agency partners have received small private grants to assist in the acquisition of educational materials, supplies, and equipment requested by the leadership and management students.

Partnerships

Partners for the wellness center originally were selected from current Department of Nursing contracted agencies. The center started in spring 2005 with one partner that served high-risk parents, but that partnership was discontinued in 2006 due to constraints in the partner agency.

The Kitchen was added as a partner in 2006. This partner is a nonprofit corporation that provides services, including living accommodations and health care, to homeless and uninsured individuals within six areas. Five of the six areas within this organization were used by CHC during 2006–2007, including a walk-in center for adolescents, a temporary-shelter home for homeless women and families, a free medical clinic serving the uninsured, an independent-living apartment complex housing low-income clients 55 years of age or older or with a diagnosed disability, and a walk-in mental health center serving primarily homeless men. In 2007, a sixth area of The Kitchen was added: the nurturing center, which serves as a day care for children of parents who are living at the temporary-housing facility.

Victory Square was added as a partner in 2007. Victory Square is part of the Victory Mission corporation, a private grant- and donation-supported housing and support organization for homeless men.

Barriers

Some agencies are not a good fit for CHC. Some agencies request services that do not meet the mission, philosophy, purpose, and goals of the nursing center without walls. Therefore, selection of appropriate partnerships has been necessary to meet the intent of CHC to maintain safe and structured environments for undergraduate students.

Lack of continuity of care becomes a huge barrier because the wellness center is available only during the academic fall and spring semesters, leaving the population without a nurse for the remainder of the time. Also, the number of students varies with enrollment, and not all students choose to have clinical experiences at the center. Typically, there are ample numbers of community-health students in the fall but a very limited number in the spring, and the numbers are the opposite for the leadership-and-management students.

Lack of funding and space is an additional barrier. Much more could be accomplished with additional money to purchase equipment, supplies, and educational materials, as well as space to store student-developed health-promotion materials and client records. The Department of Nursing is currently seeking grant funding to support CHC.

Achievements

Although CHC has not received any local, regional, or national awards, the achievements for the students and clients served cannot go unnoticed. Coalition for Healthy Communities has grown in its 3 years of existence from one site to seven sites serving a wide variety of vulnerable populations. Agencies such as local senior centers have requested to be included in CHC.

Partners have gained from a nursing presence to meet the health care needs of their populations. Individual client encounters have grown, with 1,872 assessments completed; 1,454 client or group educational sessions; and 313 referrals made during the 2007–2008 academic fall and spring semesters. Nursing students have been provided with opportunities to apply evidence-based, community-focused care in a supervised setting and to conduct research on a variety of topics. Nursing students have gained experience through assessing health care needs, using health literacy skills, developing relevant educational materials, and learning by immersion about the culture of poverty. MSU nursing graduates who have participated in CHC have frequently contacted the partner organizations to volunteer following graduation, and several students have taken positions in community health since the initiation of the center. The partner organizations eagerly await the arrival of nursing students to assist the populations whose health care needs and concerns they serve. Clients served by CHC frequently ask, "When is my nurse coming back?"

Nursing faculty have conducted research on students' perceptions of poverty, service-learning before and after their experience working at the wellness center, and the student-to-student peer mentoring. Research findings have been presented at regional and national conferences and have been accepted for publication. The CHC has been a win-win situation for the department of nursing, the faculty, the students, and the community we serve.

For more information contact:

Caroline Helton, MS, MN, RN
Missouri State University
Department of Nursing
901 South National Avenue
Springfield, MO 65897
417-836-6569
CarolineHelton@missouristate.edu

Susan Sims-Giddens, EdD, RN
Missouri State University
Department of Nursing
901 South National Avenue
Springfield, MO 65897
417-836-5398
SusanSimsGiddens@missouristate.edu

Dr. Kathryn Hope
Missouri State University
901 S. National
Springfield, MO 65897
Kathrynhope@missouristate.edu

Reference

Benner, P. (1984). *From novice to expert: Excellence and power in clinical nursing practice.* Menlo Park, CA: Addison-Wesley.

Duquesne University School of Nursing Nurse-Managed Wellness Center, Pittsburgh, Pennsylvania

Overview/Beginning Development

In 1994, faculty from the Duquesne University School of Nursing established an interdisciplinary nurse-managed wellness center (DUSON NMWC) in St. Justin Plaza, a high-rise apartment building for older adults in Mt. Washington, Pennsylvania. Subsequently, with funding from a Housing and Urban Development (HUD) Community Outreach Partnership Grant, a DUSON NMWC site was opened in 1995 in a second high-rise apartment building, K. Leroy Irvis Towers, in the Hill District. In Fall 2004, an additional full-scale wellness center site was opened in the South Side Senior Center with a grant from the Birmingham Foundation. Since then, five additional wellness center sites were established at senior centers across the city of Pittsburgh through collaboration with the Citiparks Senior *Interests* program. The most recent additions to the DUSON NMWC sites include Sylvania Place and Ormsby Manor, both of which are senior residential buildings.

Mission Statement

The mission of the Duquesne University School of Nursing Nurse-Managed Wellness Center is to provide wellness-oriented health care services to vulnerable populations. The goal is to deliver holistic and culturally competent care that promotes health, functioning, and quality of life. The Center provides opportunities for interdisciplinary care experiences, service, and research for students and faculty from the university. In all aspects of care, the uniqueness and strengths of the community and of each individual receiving care are maximized and respected. Confidentiality and awareness of each individual's rights to choose are maintained.

Services

All of the DUSON NMWC sites provide the following services:

- Blood pressure screening
- Health screening
- Functional/safety assessments
- Chair exercises
- Brown-bag medicine review days
- Nutrition-education programs
- Health-education programs

Some examples of special programs in various sites are computer classes, health fairs, annual flu shot clinics, the container garden project (in collaboration with the Greater Pittsburgh Community Food Bank and local farmers), the Walk & Win programs, the Weigh-In & Win programs, senior nutrition programs, and movie nights.

Staffing

The DUSON NMWC sites are staffed by volunteer registered nurses and advanced practice nurses, many of whom are also full-time school of nursing faculty members. The hours of operation vary from 3 to 6 hours per week. Student nurses are assigned to the DUSON NWMC throughout their clinical experiences and often volunteer time in addition to the required clinical hours.

An AmeriCorps Volunteer in Service to America (VISTA) is sought each year through the combined resources of the National Nursing Center Consortium and the Duquesne University School of Nursing. This VISTA is assigned to work on a specific project identified through feedback from the clients of the NMWC.

Population Served

The DUSON NMWC primarily serves low-income, older adults who live in the city of Pittsburgh and are aging in place. These older adults represent diverse ethnic and racial backgrounds.

Reimbursement

Because clients are not charged for services rendered, the DUSON NMWC and its special projects are sustained through volunteerism, partnerships, donations, private foundations, and grants. The DUSON NMWC has been supported and funded, as have a number of special projects, by the following:

- Duquesne University School of Nursing, which provided original support to establish the NMWC at St. Justin Plaza in 1994 and provides ongoing support of faculty to practice at all sites
- Housing and Urban Development Community Outreach Partnerships Centers Program, which provided a grant to Duquesne University in 1995 and an institutionalization grant to DUSON to establish an NMWC at K. Leroy Irvis Towers in 1996
- Christian Housing Authority; Pennsylvania Housing Finance Corporation, Arbors Management; management and staff of St. Justin Plaza and K. Leroy Irvis Towers, Hill House Senior Services
- Residents and families of St. Justin Plaza and K. Leroy Irvis Towers
- Presbyterian-University Hospital Nurses Alumni Association
- Pennsylvania Department of Health, Community-Based Health Care Assistance Program, grants for resources (Tobacco Settlement Act Grants for Resources)
- Birmingham Foundation–South Side Region Resource Grant
- Pittsburgh Citiparks, Department of Parks and Recreation, Senior *Interests* Resource Grants
- Geriatric Demonstration Project from the NNCC for a walking program
- Pennsylvania Department of Community and Economic Development grant for the NMWC at the South Side Senior Center
- Ryan Memorial Foundation Grant to fund the nursing program
- Jewish Health Care Foundation Grant to fund the Computer Literacy for Seniors Project

Partnerships

The Duquesne University School of Nursing NWMC works closely with the management of the high-rise apartment buildings in which the sites are located and with Pittsburgh Citiparks, which provides the space for the work of the NMWC in Pittsburgh neighborhoods. The Duquesne University Office of Sponsored Research provides assistance in seeking funders.

Collaboration with the Duquesne University schools of pharmacy and health sciences often provides programs for more holistic wellness. Lastly, clients are actively engaged in partnership to determine their needs and provide feedback to the NMWC staff.

Barriers

Seeking ongoing funding to sustain the wellness centers is a major barrier, as is being able to staff the centers consistently. Coordinating faculty and student clinical schedules with the academic calendar is also often a challenge. Data collection that reflects outcomes of wellness interventions and intercoder reliability related to data collection also provide a considerable challenge.

Achievements

The NMWC sponsored by Duquesne University School of Nursing received international recognition when it was awarded a 1996 Archon Award by Sigma Theta Tau International Nursing Honor Society. In 1997, the Butler County Visiting Nurses Association adopted the Duquesne University School of Nursing NMWC model and opened three NMWCs: one in high-rise apartment buildings for older adults in Butler County, one in a mall, and one in a senior center. The St. Justin Plaza NMWC was awarded a 1999 Best Practice Award by HUD Neighborhood Networks. Finally, the DUSON NMWC sites at both St. Justin Plaza and K. Leroy Irvis Towers received a Certificate of Honor from the Hospital Council of Western Pennsylvania in recognition of their excellence and impact in improving community health.

For more information contact:

Lenore (Leni) K. Resick, PhD, CRNP, FNP-BC, NP-C
Associate Professor and Director
DUSON Nurse-Managed Wellness Center
412-396-5228
resick@duq.edu

Maureen Leonardo, MN, CRNP, CNE, FNP-BC
Associate Professor and Manager, St. Justin Plaza
412-396-6539
leonardo@duq.edu

Fisher Hall
600 Forbes Avenue
Pittsburgh, PA 15282
http://www.nursing.duq.edu/ctrNMWC.html

The Harriet Rothkopf Heilbrunn B'32 Academic Nursing Center Brooklyn, New York

Agency Overview

The Harriet Rothkopf Heilbrunn B'32 Academic Nursing Center (HRHANC) of the Long Island University (Brooklyn Campus) School of Nursing opened its doors and saw its first client on December 7, 2006. The HRHANC is named for and endowed by a generous contribution from a former alumna of the University.

The Mission

In keeping with the standards of the profession, the University's mission of excellence and access, and the goals of Healthy People 2010, the mission of the HRHANC is to reduce health disparities among high-risk populations by providing accessible and affordable primary, secondary, and tertiary prevention activities, focusing on risk assessment, education, counseling, and referral for vulnerable, underserved populations in downtown Brooklyn, including the Brooklyn campus community. The HRHANC seeks to integrate student clinical experience and faculty practice in the effective provision of education, health care, and research, as determined by the needs of the community.

Population Served and Services Offered

The HRHANC is located in the wellness center of the university and provides services for faculty, staff, and students of the university, as well as the surrounding area, which is a densely populated, urban area with a high rate of poverty and many health care needs. Services provided include the following:

- Weekly blood pressure screening
- Weekly weight-loss sessions
- Health-risk assessments and counseling
- Brown-bag medicine reviews
- Quarterly mammogram screening
- Monthly HIV testing and counseling
- Online and in-person smoking-cessation program
- Healthy living for older adults (funded by the Aetna Foundation)
- Quarterly bone marrow drives (to increase the database of minorities)
- Asthma education
- Healthy Monday initiatives
- Health fairs

Hours of Service and Staffing

The HRHANC is staffed 4 days a week for a total of 20 hours. However, programs are also held days, evenings, and weekends.

Partnerships and Collaborations

The center collaborates with many of the departments and schools within the university to provide services such as asthma education. Through collaboration with other departments, classes have been held on methicillin-resistant Staphylococcus aureus (MRSA), protecting your back, and other subjects geared to the interest and needs of the community.

Funding

Although the center was opened with endowed funds, which help to maintain basic functioning, grants are another source of revenue. One such grant came from the Aetna Foundation, which helps support healthy-aging classes.

Education Opportunities

The center serves as a clinical site for community health courses, as well as for teaching projects for various courses within the program.

Strengths and Limitations

Strong support from both the dean of the school and the provost of the Brooklyn Campus is a major strength, as is the center's location in an urban setting with a multiplicity of health care needs. The geographical area served has high rates of HIV, cardiac, and respiratory problems. Finding adequate funding sources to expand services is a major burden, as is coordinating faculty and student clinical schedules within the academic calendar.

For more information contact:

Esther Levine-Brill, PhD, ANP-BC
Co-Director
Harriet Rothkopf Heilbrunn B'32 Academic Nursing Center
School of Nursing
Long Island University
Brooklyn Campus
ebrill@liu.edu
http://www.brooklyn.liu.edu/nursingcenter/

Temple Health Connection, Temple University Department of Nursing, Philadelphia, Pennsylvania

Beginning Development

In 1994, Temple University Department of Nursing, College of Health Professions, under the direction of Dr. Catherine Bevil, received an HRSA Division of Nursing grant to establish an academic nursing center. The center, known as Temple Health Connection, was always envisioned as a nurse-run, nurse-managed, comprehensive health center, with nurse practitioners inside the center providing primary care and public health nurses providing health-promotion and disease-prevention initiatives to the community. Establishing a presence behind the Temple University main campus in Norris Homes & Apartments would not have been possible without the help and guidance of Diane L. Gass, Tenant Council President.

Recently, the primary care side of the center joined Philadelphia Health Management's Federally Qualified Health Center (FQHC) and is now known as PHMC Health Connection. Temple Health Connection remains as the public health/wellness side of the partnership.

Mission Statement

The mission statement of Temple Health Connection is this: "Temple Health Connection and PHMC Health Connection together are a unique University–public health agency collaboration dedicated to improving the health of the at-risk community it serves."

Temple Health Connection is dedicated to health promotion and disease prevention. The goals of the center and its relationship with PHMC are the following:

1. Primary-care practice. The center's programs include all ages, with a significant concentration on adolescent and women's health, including contraceptive management, and safe-sex-practice education for both men and women.
2. Education for graduate and undergraduate students. PHMC provides enrichment for students from Temple as well as the surrounding universities. Temple Health Connection is invigorated by the presence of Temple nursing and public health students year round.
3. Scholarship & Research. Temple Health Connection/PHMC Health Connection Practice provides the opportunity for scholarship and projects for graduate students in the community center, as well as clinical practice. Projects have received grants and funding, for example, for pediatric studies regarding immunization. Presentations have been made at national conferences on implementation of our patient electronic record.
4. Service and Outreach. Temple Health Connection is a major effort to meet the needs of the surrounding community with funding for lead removal, teen after-school programs, and summer camps.
5. Faculty Practice. Faculty from Temple University practice at PHMC as part of their faculty "teaching."

Services

Temple Health Connection (THC) provides or has provided the following services:

- Lead-safe babies
- Asthma-safe kids
- Nurse–family partnership (the David Olds Model)
- Homework +, an after-school tutoring and life-enhancement program
- Norris kids summer camp
- Teen groups – Good Fella$ and The Girl Unit
- Health screenings
- SHINE: Transcultural health promotion in immigrant communities
- Open Airways in area elementary schools
- Flu shots in senior housing
- Student runs, Philly style
- Anti-tobacco awareness campaign and quit-smoking groups
- Breastfeeding support and outreach center

Staffing

Faculty and outreach workers, hired from the community, staff THC. Student nurses are assigned to THC initiatives in their community health rotations and often volunteer time in addition to the required clinical hours. Physical therapy, public health, recreational therapy, medical, and pharmacy students have also played a key role, as has the Student Nurse Association chapter at Temple University. In the summer, Bridging the Gaps students from all the health disciplines work in the summer camp and other environmental-health initiatives.

Population Served

Temple Health Connection primarily serves low-income families who live in north Philadelphia.

Reimbursement

Sustainability of the THC and special projects are made possible by partnerships, donations, private foundations, and grants. Over the years, THC and its special projects have been funded by the following organizations and agencies:

- Division of Nursing, Bureau of Health Professions
- Temple University
- Independence Foundation
- City of Philadelphia Childhood Lead Poisoning Prevention Program
- CIGNA Foundation
- Environmental Protection Agency
- GlaxoSmithKline
- Health Promotion Council

- Independence Blue Cross
- National Institute of Nursing Research
- The Patricia Kind Family Foundation
- Pennsylvania Department of Public Health
- Pennsylvania Department of Health
- Philadelphia Housing Authority
- Tobacco Settlement Act Grants Award for Resources
- STEPS for a Healthier Philadelphia
- National Nursing Centers Consortium
- Will & Jada Smith Family Foundation
- Southeast Pennsylvania March of Dimes
- Southeast Pennsylvania Area Health Education Center

Partnerships

- PHMC Health Connection
- National Nursing Centers Consortium
- Nurse Family Partnership Collaborative
- Penn State Integrated Pest Management
- Community Asthma Prevention Program (CAPP)
- Bridging the Gaps

Barriers

Achieving ongoing funding for sustainability is the major barrier.

Achievements

Temple Health Connection has been the recipient of several awards:

- National Environmental Education Foundation & Training (NEEFT) for Health Promotion Excellence for Lead Awareness: North Philly Style
- Southeastern PA American Lung Association award for health promotion
- GlaxoSmithKline Community IMPACT Award

Temple Health Connection was chosen as the exemplar for the Temple University Middle States visit reflecting the trifold mission of the university: education, research, and service.

For more information contact:

Rita J. Lourie, MSN, MPH, RN
610-348-9695
rlourie@temple.edu

Kathleen Mahoney, PhD, CRNP
215-707-3452
Kathleen.mahoney@temple.edu

Nancy L. Rothman, EdD, RN
Independence Foundation Chair of Urban Community Health Nursing
215-707-5436
rothman@temple.edu

Department of Nursing
College of Health Professions
Temple University
3307 N. Broad Street
Philadelphia, PA 19140

University of Delaware Nursing Center
Newark, Delaware

Agency/Program Overview

The University of Delaware Nursing Center was established in 1994 with a focus on wellness for older adults and a focus on specialty care and case management for frail, older people. At the time of initial funding from HRSA, the center proposed to support the increasing geriatric-care needs of adults and their families in northern Delaware. For more than the next 10 years, the center has provided comprehensive geriatric assessments with related case management to older Delawareans. Due to the small size of Delaware, the center is able to meet needs on a statewide basis. With changes in funding and faculty support, the center offers its services through student-outreach activities and faculty time designated for service, outreach, and scholarship. The center maintains a focus on community-dwelling older adults and has expanded to include a focus on other vulnerable populations. Vulnerable populations are identified as those groups who have significant health risks, may be underserved, and often lack the personal attributes or abilities to promote and meet their own wellness needs.

Founding Mission

The nursing center's mission is to promote the health, wellness, and quality of life of older adults and their families. As an academic nursing center, the center includes three major areas of programming: (1) service and outreach to the community, (2) education for graduate and undergraduate students, and (3) scholarship and research activities that document outcomes of faculty outreach and teaching.

Vision

The nursing center's vision is "Caring for Today and Educating for Tomorrow."
    "The test of our progress in not whether we add more to the abundance of those who have much, it is whether we provide enough for those who have little" (Franklin Delano Roosevelt, 1937).

Services Provided

Service and outreach to the community have included statewide senior peer counseling, health fairs, ongoing monthly blood pressure screenings at senior centers, comprehensive geriatric assessments, and smoking-cessation strategies targeting 18–24-year-olds. The statewide senior peer sharing has been funded with HRSA and state contracts and trains peer counselors to lead local community meetings focused on health issues for older adults, usually in senior centers. As a "center without walls," the wellness center takes services to clients in the community. Assessment times are arranged with the individual clients and/or families. Outreach activities to community groups (i.e., schools, senior centers) are planned to best meet the needs of the audience. Community events, such as wellness days and health fairs, are also scheduled. Health promotion services, most of which are funded by HRSA, have been expanded to include vulnerable older adult and Hispanic populations.

Education Opportunities

Wellness center services provide clinical opportunities for undergraduate students (traditional and accelerated programs). These opportunities have allowed for revision and enhancement of the undergraduate curriculum (with AACN-Hartford funding to support implementation of geriatric nursing care content in UD curriculum), including the development of a stand-alone nursing elective, senior leadership experiences in gerontological nursing, integration of the Omaha System into documentation content in the sophomore year, and revision of the health-promotion course to increase geriatric content. The wellness center also provides a clinical-practice learning site for clinical-nurse-specialist and nurse-practitioner students, and service-learning and volunteer opportunities for all UD nursing students.

Reimbursement

Clients are not charged for services rendered. The wellness center has been sustained through grants, donations, volunteerism, and partnerships with local agencies working to meet needs of older adults or other vulnerable populations (e.g., HRSA, AACN-Hartford, Jessie Ball DuPont, and Lung Association of Delaware). Grants have been the most useful source of financial support.

Achievements

More than 175 frail, older adults and their families were provided with comprehensive geriatric-assessment and case-management services in the last year. Through 10 years of monthly blood pressure checks and referrals at local senior centers, more than 7,200 people have been screened and referred at community events. The center also established a successful "Picture Yourself a Nurse" campaign, with more than 1,250 children served. Outcomes have been researched and analyzed, providing faculty with multiple opportunities for presentation and publication. Funded research programs have been conducted regarding tobacco cessation in young adults, including studies regarding attitudes related to smoking and cessation, "buddy system" research, and a peer-developed marketing campaign.

Barriers

The major challenge of the wellness center continues to be sustainability, especially with diminished funding resources. Changes in the school's administration have led to decreased and unstable institutional support.

For more information contact:

Evelyn R. Hayes, PhD, FNP-BC
Professor and Director, UD Nursing Center
377 McDowell Hall
250 North College Avenue
Newark, DE 19716
erhayes@udel.edu
302-831-8392
302-831-2382 (fax)

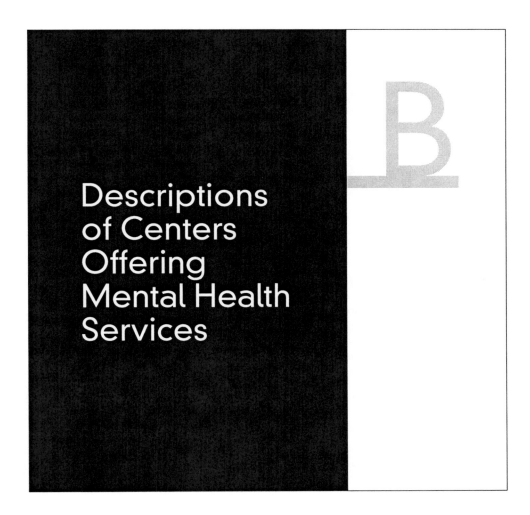

Descriptions of Centers Offering Mental Health Services

Children's Health Centers of VNA Community Services, Inc. Abington and Norristown, Pennsylvania

Agency/Program Overview

Visiting Nurse Association (VNA) Community Services, Inc., was established in 1919 to address the health and human service needs of infants, children, and families in need in eastern and central Montgomery County, Pennsylvania, and the surrounding communities. Children and families from any location are welcome.

Since the 1950s, VNA has operated traveling well-child clinics throughout the service area. In the mid-1990s, the full-service Children's Health Centers of VNA were opened in both Norristown and Abington, Montgomery County, to provide both well and sick care to children of uninsured and underinsured families. The VNA is an independent 501(c)3 organization. The Children's Health Centers of VNA are Nurse-Managed Primary Pediatric Health Care Centers.

The VNA Children's Health Centers are a support and resource for the children to whom primary pediatric care is provided. The VNA advanced practice nurses and staff do not provide mental health services directly but do understand and take the time to provide important listening and assistance with referrals and follow-up for whatever specialty services families need.

The VNA recognizes the importance of and collaborates strongly with other providers of health and social services to maximize efficient, responsive, and effective services or care.

Mission

The Mission of the VNA Community Services Children's Health Centers is, to the extent of available resources, to make quality pediatric health care services available to children whose challenging circumstances might result in their otherwise not receiving appropriate and timely routine, preventative, or emergency health care. In addition, the purpose is to provide a trusted and available "medical home" that contributes to the healthy development, school readiness, self-confidence, and success of the children served. The commitment and standard for care is that of equaling or surpassing the routine available care experienced by these children's more advantaged peers.

Goal

The goal of the VNA Community Services Children's Health Centers is to be a strong, collaborative partner and resource in a larger network of health and social service providers committed to supporting and advancing the healthy development of children and the capacity and self-confidence of their families.

Partnerships and Collaborations

VNA Community Services has formed many informal partnerships to address community needs. VNA actively cooperates and/or collaborates with the following:

- **Community or Governmental Agencies:** Children's Aid Society, Montgomery County Department of Children and Youth, Norristown Area Early Head Start, Montgomery County Head Start, Jenkintown Day Nursery, Pennsylvania Keystone Stars Program, Lakeside School for Girls, Northstar Youth Services, Carson Valley School, Saint Mary's Villa, Wordsworth Academy, Montgomery County Infant Health Advisory Council, National Nursing Center Consortium, Head Start Health Advisory Committee, Montgomery County Collaborative Board
- **Academic:** Gwynedd Mercy College, Montgomery County Community College, Villanova University, Temple University, West Chester University, Arcadia University, Jefferson University, University of Pennsylvania, Philadelphia College of Osteopathic Medicine
- **Hospitals:** Abington Memorial Hospital, Mercy Suburban General, Montgomery Hospital, Children's Hospital of Philadelphia, Saint Christopher's Hospital for Children

Service Population

The children's health centers of VNA Community Services provide services to children from birth through 21. The population that is the focus of the service is at-risk children who are without health insurance or are without a medical home. Although service focuses on children at risk because of their families' financial situations, it should be noted that 62% of the children who are seen in the centers have been diagnosed with emotional, behavioral, and/or physical disabilities.

Hours of Operation

The Abington Clinic is staffed approximately 7 hours a day, Monday through Friday. The Norristown Clinic is staffed 2 days a week with sick visits available by appointment on other weekdays. VNA also provides on-site sick and well visits once each week to children who reside in four residential facilities in our service area. Advanced practice nurses are available after hours and on weekends to respond to the health care needs of patients' families requiring immediate assistance. Families needing care for their children are encouraged to call.

Services Provided

The services provided include well and sick health care, physical examinations, developmental assessments, immunizations, home visits, and one-on-one parenting education and guidance. Additionally, VNA Community Services is able, through its Personal Navigator Program, to provide the support necessary to connect the families of the children served with 22 separate governmental and community benefits. Related VNA children's programs that improve the health and development of area children in need include Preschool Vision, Hearing and Speech Screening Program, CPR and Pediatric First Aid Program, Child Care Health Consultation Program, and educational programs for residents and staff of area residential facilities.

Current Special Initiative

A special area of interest now is participation in southeastern Pennsylvania's rollout of the Chronic Care Model for Asthma. This initiative is a comprehensive approach to improving the management of chronic illness and will utilize evidence-based change concepts to redesign care for chronic conditions, with a focus on active patient participation.

Staffing

The children's health centers of VNA Community Services are staffed with six nurse-practitioners and seven registered nurses. The children's health centers use a per diem staffing model, with the exception of one full-time nurse-practitioner, who serves as the coordinator of professional nursing services for the agency; and one part-time nurse-practitioner, who is the primary contact for residential facilities. The nurse-practitioners of the Children's Health Centers have been individually credentialed as providers for Independence Blue Cross (CHIP), Keystone Mercy, Health Partners, and Aetna. This individual credentialing strengthens the Children's Health Centers as nurse-managed centers.

Educational Opportunities

Educational opportunities are numerous. Local schools of nursing rotate students through the clinic for a portion of their pediatric experience. Nurse-practitioners precept and mentor advanced practice nursing students in both pediatrics and family practice for local Master's in Nursing programs and for physician assistance programs.

Funding

Medical Assistance, Medical Assistance HMO, CHIP, and fee for service are accepted. Grant funds and charitable donations including significant funding from the Independence Foundation and the Independence Blue Cross Charitable Medical Care Grant program and from individuals, area corporations, and local businesses. These funds ensure that no patient is turned away for an inability to pay.

Strengths and Limitations

A major strength of the Children's Health Centers is the ability to deliver high-quality primary-care services and to provide a "medical home" for at-risk children in need, while offering reassurance and guidance to parents and care-givers. VNA also values the clinical strength of its nurse-practitioners and its position as a respected health provider in Montgomery County and surrounding communities. As is the case with many nonprofit agencies, the availability of funding is a limitation and a challenge.

For more information, contact:

Lorraine Donaghy, RN
Children's Programs Practice & Operations Manager
Sue Gresko, MSN, CRNP
Coordinator, Professional Nursing Services
1421 Highland Ave.
Abington, PA 19001
215-572-7880 (phone)
215-572-8024 (fax)
http://www.vnacs.org

Second Location:
1109 Dekalb Street, Norristown, PA 19401

Eleventh Street Family Health Services of Drexel University, Philadelphia, Pennsylvania

Agency Overview

Through the leadership of Dr. Patricia Gerrity and the vision of several MCP-Hahnemann University nurses, Eleventh Street Family Health Services (Eleventh Street), a different kind of urban health care center, was formed. In 1996, several public health nursing faculty led by Dr. Gerrity asked leaders of the public housing residents' councils how the College of Nursing and Health Professions could help the community with health-related issues. Community leaders responded, "We want a place in our own neighborhood where we can get good health care and learn to stay healthy." In 1998, Dr. Gerrity received a Health Resources and Services Administration (HRSA) program grant and began delivering primary-care services to the community in offices located in a small community center connected to one of the public housing developments. Services were delivered out of this site for 4 years.

In 2002, Drexel University received $3.3 million from HRSA to build a free-standing, 17,000-square-foot "Healthy Living Center" in north Philadelphia in partnership with the Philadelphia Housing Authority. In the same year, the center formed a linkage with the Resources for Human Development Family Practice and Counseling Network, a group of federally qualified nurse-managed centers. This linkage provided higher rates of reimbursement for patients on Medicaid, and grant funds to partially subsidize the more than 30% of patients who are uninsured. Since the center opened in September 2002, the number of patients served there has grown substantially. In 2006–2007 the center's staff served patients through 20,000 visits in primary care, behavioral health, and dental care.

Mission

The goal for Eleventh Street is to provide care across the lifespan, integrating primary care and public health to address needs while building on the strengths of the community.

Center Hours and Clinical Services

Eleventh Street is open Monday through Friday and, to accommodate the increasing demand for services, the center stays open 3 evenings a week and a half day on Saturday. The center provides a range of clinical services to meet the community's self-identified needs. The holistic approach taken by Eleventh Street augments primary, behavioral, and dental care with an ever-growing menu of chronic-disease-management, health-promotion, and wellness services. The goal of Eleventh Street is to be a hub of health-related activity where patients can be treated for a variety of illnesses, and also where they can learn about healthy living and healthy eating, participate in physical fitness activities, and more. A community advisory board meets quarterly and guides services provided by Eleventh Street.

In addition to clinical areas, the clinic houses a fitness center, a teaching kitchen, and other common spaces for activities. These health-promotion activities include yoga, line dancing, self-efficacy programs, art therapy, smoking cessation, family fitness programs, and cooking classes. In response to the lack of a neighborhood grocery store, the center has partnered with the PhilAbundance food bank to provide free fresh fruit and vegetables to families each week at a local church, a long-standing partner of the health center. In collaboration with the Philadelphia Federation of Settlements, the center recently planted a garden that will be cared for and harvested by neighborhood youth, who will then sell the produce to local restaurants and to community residents. The produce will also be incorporated into the center's cooking classes for adults and teens.

The nonclinical outreach services and activities reach out to and attract people to the health center, where they learn about the full range of services available to them. Often, the activities provide an opportunity for people to come together to share health concerns and life problems. The health center has become a hub for many activities that improve the quality of life in the community.

Transdisciplinary Model of Care

At the Eleventh Street Center, staff members include the nurse-practitioners; a clinical RN; medical assistants; social workers, several of whom are embedded into primary care to address mental-health concerns; a podiatrist; a dentist and dental staff; a physical therapist; a nutritionist and health educator; front desk staff; a community-outreach worker; a van driver; and AmeriCorps members from the Philadelphia Health Corporation. The core care team is composed of a nurse-practitioner and a primary behavioral-health consultant. Depending upon each patient's needs, the team may also include a health educator/nutritionist, a physical therapist, and/or a dentist. The care team approach enables disciplines to be enriched as each provider learns from the other's role.

Using the team approach, behavioral health services are seamlessly integrated into primary care, in order to improve the effectiveness and efficiency of treatment while reducing the stigma typically associated with specialty mental health services. Essential to the practice of providers at Eleventh Street is routine screening for depression as well as the recent implementation of a trauma-informed care model to help mitigate adverse affects of traumatic life experiences on patients' overall health. Two therapists, one focused on children and the other on adults and chronic-illness management, provide behavioral consultation in primary care. Behavioral health is considered to be any behavioral factor that might affect a patient's current or future health status, broadly conceived as real or perceived, including physical health, emotional health, quality of life, and health habits. The collaboration of primary care and behavioral health strengthens the services provided to patients by placing a primary behavioral-health specialist and social worker directly in primary care.

Funding

The Eleventh Street Family Health Center is partially funded through federal, state, and private foundation grants. Through its linkage with the Family Practice and Counseling Network, Eleventh Street receives an annual grant that partially underwrites care for the uninsured as well as cost-based reimbursement for patients covered by medical assistance. Fifty-four percent of the health center's funding comes from Medical Assistance, 12% from the Pennsylvania Department of Public Welfare, 13% from U.S. Department of Health and Human Services funds, 14% from grants and donations, and 7% from other sources (e.g., patient fees, Medicare, private insurance reimbursement).

Student Experiences and Educational Opportunities

The Eleventh Street Family Health Services provides a unique opportunity for Drexel University students of all types to practice in a real-life environment. Nursing students, physical therapy students, mental health discipline students, and others practice side by side with center staff and learn how to deliver community-based care. These students see the effectiveness of transdisciplinary teams working with patients who have complex, chronic illnesses. Since the inception of Eleventh Street, over 300 RN to BSN students have been involved in health promotion activities, including making home visits, giving immunizations, teaching about diabetes, assessing seniors' homes for fall risks, and organizing community health fairs. Students receive valuable insight into the challenges and rewards of practicing as a nurse in the community setting. In addition, the School of Public Health, the College of Media Arts and Design, the College of Information Science and Technology, the College of Business, and the College of Medicine participate in the work of the health center through specific projects and programs. In late 2008, in partnership with the University's School of Law, the center will be implementing a law clinic. Services will initially target health-related matters and will grow to include a wider array of services.

Strengths and Limitations

The strengths of Eleventh Street include its transdisciplinary model and its ability to serve as an exemplary model of community-based care for faculty practice, as well as clinical experiences for students. In addition, the willingness and ability of staff at Eleventh Street to modify and add services to meet the community's needs must be acknowledged. Given Eleventh Street's success and related increase in the number of patients seen and array of programs offered, a shortcoming is the need for more space. The center is currently using a nearby community center for additional program space.

Recognition

Health Workforce Solutions, funded by the Robert Wood Johnson Foundation, selected Eleventh Street as one of the Innovative Models to be highlighted on the newly developed Web site InnovativeCareModels.com.

Future

The center plans to add family therapy through the College of Nursing and Health Professions Couples and Family Therapy Program. In addition, in response to patient requests, plans are also under way to expand the wellness center's offerings to include complementary and alternative therapies, such as energy medicine and holistic wellness counseling.

For more information, contact:

Patricia Gerrity, PhD, RN, FAAN
850 N. 11th St.
Philadelphia, PA 19123
215-769-1100 (phone)
215-769-1117 (fax)
Info@fpcn.us
http://www.fpcn.us

Family Practice & Counseling Network
Philadelphia, Pennsylvania

History and Overview

In 1991, Donna Torrisi joined Robert Fishman and Sue Heckrotte from Resources for Human Development and Dorothy Harrell from the Abbottsford Homes to discuss a partnership that resulted in a health center on-site in this public housing development. Ms. Torrisi and Ms. Heckrotte wrote the grant that was funded as a federally qualified health center (FQHC) through the U.S. Health Resources Service Administration (HRSA) in the first year of its FQHC funding for public housing residents. Ms. Torrisi was selected as the director, and the health center facility was created from three apartments and opened in July 1992. Seven hundred residents were served the first year. Services included primary care, behavioral health, and numerous health-education programs.

The Family Practice and Counseling Network (FPCN) has grown steadily. In 1994, an HRSA expansion grant was awarded and a second site was opened in another public housing community. In 2002, the FPCN formed a partnership with Drexel University and opened a new health center in a building operated by the university in a densely populated public housing area in North Philadelphia. With a third expansion grant in 2003, the FPCN took control of a health center in southwest Philadelphia that had been founded by the University of Pennsylvania School of Nursing. In 2004, dental services were added to one site, and these were expanded to a second site in 2008. Recently, two of the smaller centers merged into one and the Southwest Health Annex moved into a larger space, so the network now has 22 examination rooms. In 2007, the network served 10,600 patients in 44,000 visits. Over 80% of the patients are of African American descent and two thirds are female.

Mission

The mission of the Family Practice and Counseling Network is this: "The Health Centers exist to provide quality, comprehensive health services to all the people they serve with special attention to vulnerable people and residents of public housing communities." The following beliefs support the network's mission:

- Quality health care is a right, not a privilege. No one will be turned away because of inability to pay.
- Health centers work best when they are partnerships between consumers and staff.
- Health education is vital to empower individuals to make choices about their health.

Health Center Services

FQHC services include primary care for all ages, prenatal care, family planning, behavioral health, and oral health care. These services are provided by a culturally competent and sensitive staff in an emotionally safe environment. In addition to these services, the FPCN strives to provide patients with education, encouragement, and assistance to self-manage their illnesses. It also provides services that support its patients' bodies, minds, and spirits, and that support them in functioning at their highest level. Some of these wellness services include these:

- Diabetic Education—A certified diabetic educator meets one-on-one and in groups with diabetic patients to coach them on self-care and addressing barriers to health.
- Cancer Support—A social worker provides a haven for patients and families to share struggles, fears, and triumphs as they live with cancer.
- Breast Health—This program provides health education, breast exams, and mammograms to women over the age of 40.
- Men's Wellness—This program provides outreach and a men's clinic within the clinic.
- G.I.R.L.S. (Gaining Independence Rebuilding Lives Successfully)—This program addresses issues on growing up female, including date rape and self-esteem.
- Peaceful Posse—This program is led by trained leaders using a rigorous curriculum that addresses issues of violence, affording boys the opportunity for health after experiences as victims, witnesses, or perpetrators. It also challenges the culture of revenge. It is built on the principle "hurt people hurt people."
- Teens Making a Difference—This program works to enhance life skills for youth, including helping with college applications and funding opportunities. A group leader who grew up in the projects and built a successful career, working her way out of poverty, serves as a role model.
- Reach Out and Read—This nationally acclaimed literacy program provides a new book for children ages 6 months to 5 years at well-child visits, as well as education for the primary care provider about the value of reading to children.
- Lead Safe Babies—Outreach workers make home visits to educate parents about lead and assess levels in patients' homes.
- Asthma Safe Kids—Outreach workers make home visits to educate children and parents about asthma prevention and care.
- Substance Abuse Recovery—An outreach worker who herself is in recovery facilitates a support group.
- Bridging the Gaps—Health students in medicine, nursing, and dental provide services to the community in a summer program.
- Welfare to Work—Welfare recipients are afforded work experiences within the health centers, with opportunities for hire.
- Nurse-Family Partnership—Patients in their first pregnancy are referred to this program for intensive case management by an RN. The program can last through the second year of the baby's life.

Future Plans for Wellness Programs

The FPCN plans to expand the one-on-one mindfulness meditation that is currently used successfully by one mental health therapist to larger numbers of patients and staff by establishing groups.

Hours and Staffing

The FPCN is open from 9:00 a.m. until 7:00 p.m. daily except Fridays, and on Saturdays from 9:00 a.m. until 1:00 p.m. Nurse-practitioners provide most FPCN primary health services, but patients have the benefit of services of a team of culturally sensitive staff, with people from the community that is being served when possible. The team includes nurses, medical assistants, psychologists, psychiatrists, social workers, outreach workers, dentists, dental hygienists and assistants, and a physician who provides prenatal care. Other staff include escorts, van drivers, and receptionists.

Partnerships and Collaborations

Partnerships are vital to the provision of services and include the National Nursing Centers Consortium, the Independence Foundation, Independence Blue Cross, Cigna Corporation, Drexel University, Family Planning Council, Bridging the Gaps, Physicians for Social Responsibility, the Wellness Community, the Susan G. Komen Breast Cancer Foundation, Reach Out and Read, the Health Federation of Philadelphia, the State Department of Health, the Pennsylvania Association of Community Health Centers, and the Department of Public Welfare.

Recognitions

The FPCN has received many awards, including the Smith Kline Beecham Community Impact Award, the National HRSA Models That Work Award, and the Health Strategy Network Award. Additionally, the director has received awards from Villanova University, the University of Pennsylvania, and the Pennsylvania State Nurses Association.

Funding

The FPCN is a Federally Qualified Health Center, so its largest source of funding is cost-based reimbursement for Medicaid visits. It also has malpractice coverage through the Federal Tort Claim Act. The Network receives a $1.5 million HRSA grant and numerous smaller grants from foundations, such as the Independence Foundation, Independence Blue Cross, and Cigna Corporation. Additionally, fees from Medicare, private insurers, and patients' fees help make up the more than $8 million budget.

For more information, contact:

Donna L. Torrisi, MSN, CRNP
Network Executive Director
Family Practice & Counseling Network
4700 Wissahickon Ave.
Philadelphia, PA 19144
267-597-3601
donna@rhd.org
http://www.fpcn.us

Health Resource Center of Cincinnati, Inc., Cincinnati, Ohio

Agency/Program Overview

The Health Resource Center of Cincinnati, Inc. (HRC) was opened in 1995 as a free, nurse-managed clinic, which was part of a faculty practice plan at the College of Nursing, University of Cincinnati. In 2000, the agency became an independent 501(c)3 entity affiliated with the College of Nursing through the president and CEO, Connie Wilson, who was a professor of nursing and a licensed independent counselor. Her release time was paid for by a professorship in psychiatric nursing grant from the Ohio Department of Mental Health.

Mission

HRC's mission is to serve the homeless and at-risk individuals who are in need of medical, psychiatric, or social services and whose needs are not being met by other agencies.

Partnerships and Collaborations

Connections to other agencies include contracts with the Hamilton County Mental Health and Recovery Services Board, Cincinnati Health Care for the Homeless, and the Adult Parole Authority. Collaborations are also in place with the Free Store Food Bank; IKRON, a behavioral health and psych rehabilitation employment service; Prospect House, a residential treatment center for men; and all of the university clinics and multiple city agencies that work with the homeless population.

Service Population and Hours

The focus of services offered is on the indigent and homeless, mentally ill people (age 18 and over) in Cincinnati, especially those who do not meet the criteria for Medicaid. An additional focus has centered upon newly released felons and sex offenders. The HRC has been instrumental in the development of two agencies in the city: Anthony House, a drop-in center for homeless adolescents; and Cincinnati Respite Center, a 24-hour facility for medically sick homeless persons. The hours of service are Monday through Thursday from 9 a.m. until 3 p.m. Clinic staff members are available on Fridays so that people can pick up prescriptions if needed. There is a 24-hour call system available for clients as well as other agencies.

Services Provided

Individual services offered include the following:

- Medical (physical exams, laboratory services, medications, and chronic care treatment)
- Behavioral health (diagnostic assessments, pharmacotherapy, medication management, and individual counseling)

- Substance-abuse services (assessments, outpatient interventions, referrals to inpatient and detoxification services, medication management, and counseling)
- Prevention (HIV, TB, and pregnancy screenings) and wellness services (psycho education)

HRC fills the service gap for persons not treated at other agencies because of the need that most agencies have to treat only those people for whom reimbursement is available. The HRC treats those who cannot access services elsewhere.

Staffing

The staff configuration includes four advanced practice registered nurses (two full-time CNSs, one full-time NP, and one part-time CNS/NP), two licensed counselors (one full-time, one part-time), and one physician, two psychiatrists, and two family practice/psychiatric residents (all part-time). Office staff includes a director of development, an intake worker, and Medicaid support staff (all full-time). The past director supervises the counseling interns and consults with clinic staff.

Funding

Funding is primarily from donations and fundraising activities, but other sources include grants and contracts and reimbursements from Medicaid for a small part (20%) of the population. Most medications are free to patients, with some requiring a small co-pay. Services and medications are fully provided if the person does not have the ability to pay.

Strengths and Limitations

Much of the HRC's strength comes from having secured certification from the Ohio Department of Mental Health and the Ohio Department of Alcohol and Drug Addiction Services, and 3-year accreditation from the Council on Accreditation of Rehabilitation Facilities (CARF). Additional strengths include the multidisciplinary aspect of care and the integration of medical, psychiatric, and substance-abuse services in one location. Counseling services offered at no charge are a draw for consumers who only receive case management services in other city agencies. Limitations include funding, which is a perennial issue; space, because the clinic exists in one large room inside the Free Store Food Bank; and the need for recognition as a viable entity by competing agencies that are bigger and much better funded.

Educational Opportunities

Educational opportunities abound because the clinic was opened with the focus of multidisciplinary education from day one and was the primary reason that the CEO received the ODMH grant for release time. Residents and counseling interns remain for 1 year, nursing students rotate through on a quarter or semester time frame, and medical students come for a period of 1 month.

All students learn to work with other disciplines and learn the strengths and limitations of each. Most have described the experience as the most fruitful of their entire career.

Evidenced-based practice is the main component of the student experience and is the focus of the certifying agencies. **Advocacy** toward improving the health of all citizens, insured or uninsured, is an underlying philosophy. No student or staff person leaves the agency without a better understanding of that philosophy and without having done his or her part in improving the life of a homeless or indigent person.

For more information, contact:

Mary Elizabeth Earle, RN, CNS
112 E. Liberty Street
Cincinnati, OH 45202
513-357-4602 (phone)
513-357-4696 (fax)
http://www.hrcci.org

Integrated Health Care, Chicago, IL

Agency Overview

Integrated Health Care (IHC) is an academic, nurse-managed center of the University of Illinois at Chicago College of Nursing (UIC CON). Since 1998, the College of Nursing has partnered with Thresholds Psychiatric Rehabilitation Centers to provide integrated primary health care to their clients (called members) with serious mental illnesses (SMI) by locating primary care clinics in existing Thresholds centers. Thresholds is the largest and oldest provider of psychiatric rehabilitation and recovery services in Illinois. At the three IHC clinic sites, CON faculty family nurse practitioners (FNPs) provide primary health care service to clients who have or are at risk for co-morbid chronic disease, in collaboration with Thresholds staff who provide mental health services.

The IHC model provides more than side-by-side delivery of primary and mental health services because the care itself is integrated (McDevitt, Braun, Noyes, Snyder & Marion, 2005). The FNPs incorporate additional skills and knowledge, such as cognitive-behavioral techniques, in the delivery of primary care services. FNPs regularly consult with faculty psychiatric mental health advanced practice nurses (PMH APNs) and also engage in joint educational programs, grand rounds, and case studies with Thresholds staff. These activities provide cross-training and facilitate creative care planning through which best practices emerge.

Mission

The mission of Integrated Health Care is to provide high-quality advanced practice nursing care to address together the primary and mental health needs of individuals with severe mental illness. This health care model promotes education, research, and dedication to professional and community collaboration.

Partnerships and Collaboration

IHC has enjoyed a long-standing partnership with Thresholds Rehabilitation Centers. In 2007, IHC entered a partnership with Mile Square Health Center of the University of Illinois Chicago Medical Center, which brought IHC under the umbrella of a Federal Qualified Health Center (FQHC). IHC also collaborates with community agencies, pharmacies, UIC departments, CON faculty, and physicians. IHC is an active participant in many professional organizations, including but not limited to the National Nursing Center Consortium, the American Public Health Association, and the National Organization for Nurse Practitioner Faculties.

Services Provided

The services provided include annual comprehensive history and physical examinations; management of acute and chronic diseases; and preventive services such as vaccinations, and screenings for diabetes, blood pressure, and cholesterol. Using evidence-based practice guidelines, FNPs monitor laboratory results, prescribe medications, and provide education to promote healthy lifestyles.

In addition, FNPs provide expanded service to Thresholds members enrolled in special programs, including the Lauren Juhl Young Adult Center, and mothers and children enrolled in the Thresholds Mothers Project. These additional services include screening and referrals for eating disorders and counseling on child care, family planning, sexual health, and other lifestyle issues.

Hours of Operation

IHC North and South are open Monday through Friday, 9 a.m.–5 p.m. The Mothers clinic is open 2 days per week. The clinics provide on-call coverage 24 hours per day, 7 days per week.

Staffing

IHC is staffed by seven family nurse-practitioners (four FTEs), one psychiatric nurse clinical specialist, one registered nurse, two medical assistants, and two nurses in management positions. All faculty are master's prepared and function as preceptors for pre-licensure and graduate nursing students who rotate through the clinics.

Funding

IHC is funded by fee-for-service reimbursement, grants, and private donations, and offers a sliding-fee discount for uninsured members. In 2007, IHC was awarded FQHC status through Mile Square Health Centers of the University of Illinois Chicago Medical Center. FQHC status provides higher Medicaid reimbursement rates. Also, in 2007, IHC was awarded a 5-year, $1.9 million HRSA grant to fund an innovative outreach program called IHC Without Walls (WOW).

Strengths and Limitations

IHC strengths include a focus on innovation, quality, and financial sustainability. In 2001, the program received the Innovation in Health Care Access Award from the Illinois Nurses Association. In 2004, IHC was chosen as an exemplar model of integrated primary and mental health service by the Bazelon Center for Mental Health Law. The program consistently receives high member satisfaction scores. Member satisfaction is further evidenced by the increasing utilization of clinic services, from 200 member visits in 1998 to over 4,000 visits in 2007. In addition, quality is measured through chart audits, which demonstrate a high rate of nurse-practitioner adherence to evidence-based primary care guidelines. IHC has achieved financial sustainability through dedicated efforts that include grant awards, partnerships, and a focus on good business practices.

IHC limitations might better be viewed as program challenges. FQHC status was achieved through a partnership resulting in somewhat diminished College of Nursing control over IHC operations. In addition, FQHC status required significant structure and equipment changes and higher-than-expected transition expenses. A lack of effective systems for coordination of services between IHC and Thresholds staff continues to be a challenge to efficient communication. Future planning will address team functioning and coordination of care.

Educational Opportunities

IHC offers rich educational opportunities for pre-licensure and advanced practice nursing students, as well as College of Nursing faculty, who rotate through all the clinic sites.

Current Special Initiative

The IHC focus for the future is on the implementation of IHC WOW. This outreach program will bring IHC's integrated model of primary and mental health service to the community in the form of nurse-practitioner house calls, group medical visits, and telemonitoring. IHC WOW will serve members who have or are at risk for chronic illness and who, by nature of their mental illness, are unable to leave home. The program also plans to enhance student and faculty learning and experiences relative to integrated primary and mental health services.

For more information, contact:

Emily Brigell, MS, RN
Director of Integrated Health Care
312-996-9354 (phone)
312-996-7725 (fax)
South: 734 W. 47 St., Chicago, IL 60609
North: 4219 N. Lincoln, Chicago, IL 60618
Mothers: 1110 W. Belmont, Chicago, IL 60657
http://www.uic.edu/nursing/pma/services/ihc/

McAuley Health Center
Detroit, Michigan

Agency Overview

The McAuley Health Center is a nurse-managed health care center that opened in 2002. The center is an independent 501(c)3 academic nursing center and is affiliated with the University of Detroit Mercy. The center was the first nurse-managed center in Detroit, and it has grown to handle nearly 3,000 patient visits a year. The center was funded by an HRSA grant and focused on the uninsured, but it now accepts both uninsured and insured patients.

Mission

The center's work is reflective of the mission of the university, which is to provide excellent, student-centered undergraduate and graduate education in an urban context. The integration of the intellectual, spiritual, ethical, and social development of students is the highest priority. In addition, the center provides opportunities for faculty practice and provides mental health services on-site.

Population Served and Services Offered

McAuley Health Center primarily provides services to underserved, migrant, and homeless, predominantly adult, African American community members on Detroit's east side. Services offered on-site include medical care (physical examinations); behavioral health assessment and treatment; substance-abuse treatment; urgent and medical care; health promotion and health education; and individual, group, and marital therapy.

Hours of Service

McAuley Health Center is open Monday through Friday, 8:30 a.m.–5:00 p.m. Both scheduled and same-day appointments are available.

Staffing

At McAuley Health Center, there are three full-time certified primary care nurse-practitioners, one full-time medical assistant, one full-time administrative assistant, one half-time biller, one project director (70%), and one part-time psychiatric mental health nurse-practitioner who is board certified (PMHNP-BC). These staff are assisted by graduate and undergraduate nursing students.

Collaborators

McAuley Health partners and collaborators include the University of Detroit College of Nursing, Mercy's College of Health Professions, and the McAuley School of Nursing, as well as the Mercy Primary Care Center (a unit of Trinity Health).

Connections to Other Agencies and Payment Resources

Referrals are made to the University of Detroit Mercy Counseling Center, where students and faculty from the university's Counseling and Addiction Studies Program work with clients. In addition, clients are referred to the PMHNP-BC if uninsured. Medicare, Medicaid, HMOs, fee for service, and Blue Cross-Blue Shield are the primary resources for payment.

Strengths and Limitations

McAuley Health Center has become a trusted community partner in providing high-quality primary care services to an underserved population. A challenge for McAuley is to establish equitable reimbursement from health plans and to establish more steady revenue streams.

Educational Opportunities for Students

McAuley provides practice for students in undergraduate nursing (bachelor's degree and accelerated second bachelor's degree), family nurse-practitioner (master's degree), counseling and addiction studies (master's degree), health systems management (master's degree or certificate) and health services administration (master's degree).

Advocacy or Future Focus

In the future, McAuley plans to provide services to children.

For more information, contact:

Carla J. Groh, PhD, PMHNP-BC
5555 Conner Ave., Suite 2691
Detroit, MI 48213
313-579-1182 (phone)
313-579-5128 (fax)
http://healthprofessions.udmercy.edu/mcauley-health-center/index.htm

University of St. Francis Health and Wellness Center
Joliet, Illinois

Agency/Program Overview

The Health and Wellness Center (HWC) is an academically affiliated nurse-managed center in downtown Joliet, Illinois. It was founded by the University of St. Francis College of Nursing and Allied Health and opened in January 2007. The HWC was designated an Edge Runner by the American Academy of Nurses Raise the Voice campaign to transform America's health care system in 2008, for developing a "nurse-driven" model of integrated primary physical and mental health care and interventions.

Mission

The mission of the University of St. Francis Health and Wellness Clinic is threefold:

- Improve access to primary health and wellness care
- Educate nursing students (undergraduate and graduate) in the delivery of community-based primary care
- Provide interdisciplinary educational experiences (Social work, special education, recreation administration, accounting, business management, marketing, and foreign languages students will be involved with the center.)

Partnerships and Collaborations

The HWC's main clinic is in a Joliet Housing Authority building, and there is a satellite clinic that provides primary health care and mental health services to Groundwork Domestic Violence Shelter for women and their children in Joliet two days per week. The main clinic has referral agreements with the Will Grundy Free Clinic, Cornerstone Services for people with disabilities, Stepping Stones Recovery Center, and Will County Health Department. It contracts with the Will County Community Health Program (WCCHP) to provide STD clinic services as a WCCHP satellite site. The HWC is the central element in a collaboration-of-care partnership and has received unprecedented support from the community. The collaboration includes the above agencies plus Catholic Charities, Joliet Public Schools District 86, Lamb's Fold Women's Center, Provena Saint Joseph Medical Center, Senior Services Center of Will County, Silver Cross Hospital, and United Way of Will County. By bringing together providers and consumers through this effort, this collaboration will collectively expand the coordination and provision of health and wellness services to underserved populations in the community.

Service Population

The HWC's patient base is the place-bound elderly and disabled, victims of domestic violence, the working poor, and the uninsured. The most common reasons for a visit are hypertension, depression, hyperlipidemia, diabetes, and routine physicals.

Services Provided

Services provided include chronic disease management, well baby and well child examinations, school and sports physicals, women's health counseling, breast exams, hypertension and diabetes mellitus screenings, asthma screenings, immunizations, flu shots, parenting education, exercise classes, grief counseling, diet and nutrition counseling, and episodic illness care. The HWC also provides psychotherapy, health promotion and education, on-site social work services, prescriptive services, and medication monitoring.

Hours of Operation

The HWC allows time for walk-ins as well as scheduled appointments, and provides evening hours to increase accessibility. The HWC is open Mondays, 8 a.m.–4 p.m.; Tuesdays, 11 a.m.–6 p.m.; Wednesdays, 9 a.m.–4 p.m.; Thursdays, 11 a.m.–6 p.m.; and Fridays (satellite clinic only), 9 a.m.–noon.

Staffing

HWC providers use a collaborative team approach. The staff configuration includes the center director, who is an FNP (full-time); three FNPs, one ANP, and one CNS (all part-time); a medical assistant (full-time); a social worker (part-time); a nursing assistant (full-time); an administrative assistant (full-time); and a student nurse. These providers use a collaborative team approach to do the following: (1) improve access to quality primary health care services to the poor and uninsured in Will County, particularly the greater Joliet area; and (2) develop and implement a model of nurse-managed primary health care that integrates both physical and mental health assessment, treatment, and follow-up services.

Funding

HWC patients without insurance pay on a sliding scale based on their income. Special fee arrangements are made for residents of local homeless and domestic violence shelters. The University of St. Francis Health and Wellness Center is an HRSA grantee ($2.1 million grant award 1D11HP07363-01-00, July 2006–June 2011). The long-term goal for the HWC, however, is financial sustainability. Toward that end, the HWC has become a recognized Blue Cross and Blue Shield, United Healthcare, Medicare, and Medicaid provider. It receives 8% of its income from private insurance, 3% from Medicare, 44% from cash payment, and 30% from the Illinois Department of Public Aid. Fifteen percent of the care provided goes without charge to residents in the local homeless and domestic violence shelters.

Strengths and Limitations

The HWC was founded and is managed by a team of advanced practice nurses—nurse-practitioners and clinical nurse specialists—who, through weekly team meetings, provide input and share perspectives on case management and approaches to care. The strengths of the HWC include the integration of mental and physical health services in the program and at both locations. There is a psychiatric mental health clinical nurse specialist embedded at the HWC who provides follow-up on mental health screenings, on-site psychotherapy, psychiatric evaluations and assessments, prescriptive services, and consultation and medication monitoring services. A social worker is also embedded in the program to offer a full array of social services to referred patients. This provides a one-stop shopping approach to comprehensive health care for individuals who have few resources and scant access to transportation and funds. One HWC provider writes a monthly health-promotion and education column in the Joliet Housing Authority newsletter, which reaches over 900 units/families in the housing complex. The most compelling challenges currently faced are securing sufficient funding for the long term, securing and coordinating specialty referrals for the uninsured and those with Medicaid, and optimizing the staffing mix to best serve the target population.

Educational Opportunities

The HWC is a clinical site for undergraduate and graduate nursing and social work student practicum and clinical rotations. Staff providers also serve as preceptors for these students.

For more information, contact:

Mary Maragos, MS, APN, CNP
Center Director
Carol Wilson, PhD, APN, CNP
Project Director
Deena Nardi, PhD, APN, CNS, FAAN
Co-Project Director
John C. Murphy Building
311 N. Ottawa St.
Joliet, IL 60432
815-774-9037
http://www.stfrancis.edu/hwc/

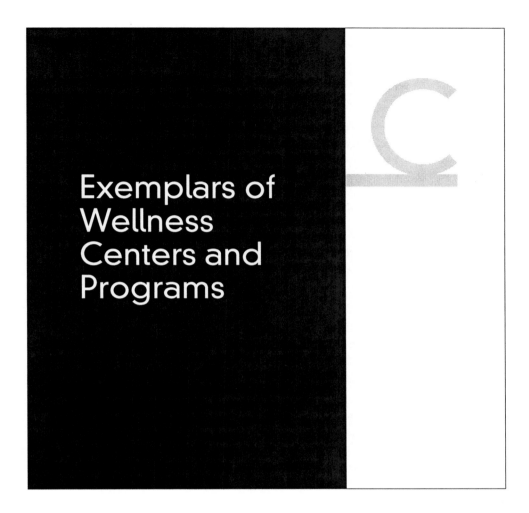

Exemplars of Wellness Centers and Programs

La Salle Neighborhood Nursing Center
Philadelphia, Pennsylvania

Ana Catanzaro, PhD, RN

Sharon Starr, MSN, RN

La Salle Neighborhood Nursing Center is a community-based nurse-managed wellness center affiliated with La Salle University's School of Nursing and Health Sciences. The center has a 16-year history of providing community-centered public health nursing and social services to at-risk, underserved populations in the southeastern Pennsylvania region. The goal of the La Salle Neighborhood Nursing Center is to improve the health of individuals, families, and communities. Its mission is to support and enhance the teaching, learning, and service mission of the School of Nursing and Health Sciences. La Salle Neighborhood Nursing Center provides diverse public health services through multiple funded and unfunded programs.

La Salle Neighborhood Nursing Center began in 1991 as a clinical laboratory for nursing students for their public health rotation. In response to community invitation, the nursing center was located in a community building that also housed a local early-learning center. Although La Salle Neighborhood Nursing Center has physically moved to various neighborhood venues, including a YWCA and a low-income housing center, throughout its 16-year history, the offices currently reside on the La Salle University campus. The staff members maintain their services mostly in the communities with the populations that they serve. The nursing center has responded to the needs of populations in Philadelphia and Bucks counties and has expanded through key partnerships into all five counties of the southeastern Pennsylvania region. This overview will highlight the programming and staffing that makes La Salle Neighborhood Nursing Center a unique and vibrant wellness center.

Programs

Health Intervention Program

La Salle Neighborhood Nursing Center provides services to a variety of populations mostly in urban settings. The first funded program was a perinatal home-visiting program providing family-centered health and social services through Philadelphia Department of Public Health Division of Maternal, Child and Family Health with Title V funding. That early home-visiting program evolved into the Health Intervention Program (HIP) for Families, which serves families in which there is a child with special health care needs. La Salle's HIP for Families team of five enrolled 170 families last fiscal year. The team includes two public health nurses, a counselor, a social worker, and a community health worker. Two team members are bilingual in Spanish and English. Families experience many challenges in raising their growing children, and it is the purpose of this program to assist families with children with special needs to live as much as possible a life similar to that of typically developing children.

Children and their families present to HIP for Families with multiple health risks. The children's health risks may include prematurity of birth; neurological, cardiac, respiratory, gastrointestinal, nutritional, metabolic, and endocrine disorders; and developmental delays and mental illness. The HIP for Families team discovered that more than half of the parents of the special needs children also experienced significant physical and/or mental health compromises that influenced their daily care of their children. Interventions provided by the HIP for Families team include those identified by the Minnesota Department of Public Health, Section on Public Health Nursing. These include outreach, screening, referral and follow-up, case management, delegation of functions, health teaching, counseling, consultation, collaboration, coalition building, community organizing, and advocacy. Interventions with and on behalf of the clients occur with various community resources and resource people, including those from schools, welfare, Social Security, hospitals and clinics; early interventionists; legal aid; and public health providers. Staff promote family relationships with community resource people and advocate with the parents to obtain necessary resources.

The HIP for Families team has found many critical urban barriers that inhibit healthy living. Affordable housing and employment opportunities are two such challenges. Many families are unable to find appropriate, affordable housing. The old housing stock is often inappropriate for the health and safety of children, especially those with special health care needs. Many families live in crowded and overwhelmingly unhealthy conditions because they cannot afford to move. Sustaining special-health children in a shelter or in transitional housing can hinder the health maintenance and welfare of that susceptible child. When a family lives in a shelter, finding alternatives for siblings when one child is hospitalized often opposes the rules that the shelter sets, leading to rejection from the shelter. Housing is a critical impasse for families with a child who has special needs. Clients welcome the chance to work, only to find that they cannot maintain their job because of transportation, child care, and child health needs. Lack of child care and the nature of their children's immediate needs often impose fluctuations in attending work or school, resulting in subsequent job losses.

Philadelphia Park Racetrack

In 1995, La Salle Neighborhood Nursing Center received an invitation from the community chaplain to provide nursing triage and care to the horsemen and horsewomen of the backstretch of Philadelphia Park Racetrack. As with perinatal home visiting, the nursing students were the first to pilot this program, followed by a community grant for a men's health initiative. The program continues and is currently funded by the Philadelphia Thoroughbred Horsemen's Association at the racetrack. The human population of Philadelphia Park consists of 1,000 men and women who work with the horses of the racetrack, including nearly 200 people who live in the dormitories close to the horse barns. Although Philadelphia Park is open all year, the horsemen and horsewomen come and go from the park in their service to the horses that race in various venues throughout the year. The population is mostly male, mostly Hispanic, with an age range of 18 to 70 years. The mean age is 40 years old. The job these men and women do is very demanding physically. They are confronted with large animals that bite, kick, and pull against human frames. Additionally, they are at risk nutritionally because backstretch residents do not have cooking privileges and rely on a small café for their food. Their work schedules of early hours to midday, followed by late-day activity, allows for boredom, loneliness, and time for behavioral health risks of tobacco, drug, and alcohol use. The chemicals in their environment put them at risk for toxicities. The horsemen and horsewomen are often uninsured as a result of their immigrant status and mobility between states.

The La Salle Nursing Center provides a 3-hour weekly session during the horsemen and horsewomen's first break of the day. The goal for staffing this center is to find a nurse who can be consistent throughout the year and to include nursing students at the weekly sessions. It is important that at least one of the backstretch nurses be bilingual, but that a uniquely qualified person sometimes is hard to find for this interval of work. Nursing center logs show more than 1,000 encounters annually, with about 30 encounters during each weekly session. Nurses administered 140 influenza, pneumonia, and tetanus vaccinations last year.

In addition to weekly blood pressure and weight screenings, the nursing center operates a laboratory for screening of blood glucose and cholesterol monitoring. The nurses offer these screenings with health education and referral to primary care for supportive diagnosis and treatment. Students organize an annual health fair that connects the horsemen and horsewomen with community vendors for health, safety, and family supports. A volunteer physician collaborates with the nursing center staff by providing medical and prescription resources. The horsemen and horsewomen stop in to thank the nurses for their assistance in recognizing and referring health issues to appropriate medical resources. The La Salle student nurses repeatedly request this clinical experience and value their work with the backstretch population.

Bristol Senior Center

La Salle Neighborhood Nursing Center maintains a practice with the elderly at the Bristol Senior Center in Bucks County. The nursing center's Lia van Rijswijk, MSN, has collaborated with the Bristol Senior Center, and the Area Agency on Aging and has also used grants from Pennsylvania Department of Community and Economic Development, Sanofi-Adventis, Proctor and Gamble, and Independence Blue Cross to provide services for the elderly. Staff, faculty, and students provide health screenings, health education and counseling, and foot care at this site. During the past year, LSNNC provided foot care to 29 seniors, counseling to 150 fracture-risk-screening participants, blood pressure screenings to 260 people (six were found to have uncontrolled hypertension and were referred for medical follow-up), medication-related health education to 29 seniors, medical referrals when indicated, and health education to 200 participating health coordinators and staff.

Child Care Health Consultation

Child care health consultation is a new service offered through La Salle Neighborhood Nursing Center. This is the practice of health professionals of promoting the health of children in early education programs, and professional staff and parents involved in the programs (American Academy of Pediatrics, American Public Health Association, National Resource Center for Health and Safety in Child Care, 2002). Professional child care staff have limited training in promoting physical, mental, social, nutritional, and oral health and safety, and in the supportive skills and knowledge needed to support children with developmental disabilities. The child care health consultant (CCHC) serves as an integral health liaison for professional early-learning-program staff in early learning centers. This relationship is built on the individual needs of the early learning center. The CCHC role is recognized nationally as a health professional role and is federally funded in the Healthy Child Care Network Support Center (Hcccnsc.edc.org). In Pennsylvania, child care health consultation was instituted through the efforts of the Pennsylvania American Academy of Pediatrics as the Early Childhood Education Linkage System. This system is responsible for providing technical assistance, and it evolved as the Healthy Childcare PA agency (Ecels-HealthyChildcarePA.org).

Health consultation is known to benefit children and their families by encouraging early education centers to reach national child care goals. Although state licensure is necessary for practice, the national and statewide goals surpass the minimum standards for the nurturing of child development based on health, growth, and unique characteristics of the individual child. Many of the national and statewide goals are health focused and require specialty professional development for goal attainment. In 2006, child care health consultation became an accreditation requirement for the National Association for the Education of Young Children. In 2006–07, at the urging of the Pennsylvania Academy of Pediatrics, the Pennsylvania Key allocated small grants to each of their regional entities for child care health consultation. However, the Pennsylvania Keystone Stars, which is sponsored by the Department of Public Welfare's Office of Child Development, provides a quality-improvement program that promotes staff education, staff participation in ongoing professional development, use of a curriculum in early learning centers; and helps practitioners support children's early learning and development. The Southeast Regional Key has expanded on quality in child care with a grant-funded position for a child care health consultant. In June 2007, La Salle Neighborhood Nursing Center (LSNNC) partnered with the regional key to provide a child care health consultant, Maryellen Malak Madden, BSN, for the five-county region.

Another advantage of this program is that La Salle Nursing undergraduate and graduate student nurses in public health nursing clinical courses who implement these services gain a greater understanding of the early education populations. Students provide local child care centers with anthropometric, vision, and hearing screenings and health promotion activities. In 2006, Dr. Zane Robinson Wolf, PhD, RN, FAAN, dean of La Salle School of Nursing and Health Sciences; Mary Ellen Miller, MSN, RN, associate director of public health programs; and the Early Childhood Education Linkage System supported Sharon Starr, MSN, RN, to become a child care health consultant trainer through the National Training Institute for Child Care Health Consultants at the University of North Carolina.

LSNNC staff, faculty, students, and volunteers provide community education, outreach, and screening services throughout the year, with nearly 800 encounters in 23 venues in the past year. These services at health fairs and community-education venues are mainly unfunded, but they provide connections with community leadership and community members for outreach of current programs and development of new initiatives.

Service Learning & Student Engagement—"Neat Feet"

Mary Ellen Miller, PhD, RN

Community Service and Learning (CSL) is required in six urban health electives at the School of Nursing and Health Sciences (SONHS) in southeastern Pennsylvania. Master's-prepared nursing staff from the wellness center are also employed as adjunct faculty members at the SONHS and are assigned to teach these particular courses. CSL activities in one course, Urban Health: Families in Jeopardy, are described below.

In this course, the impact of social, cultural, economic, and educational factors on the well-being of urban families is investigated. This elective is cross-referenced as a graduate and undergraduate course. Graduate students must complete an additional assignment, a scholarly paper that includes a community needs assessment. Both graduate and undergraduate students must engage in at least one CSL activity, minimally four hours long, as a course requirement. This requirement is stated on the course syllabus.

At the beginning of the semester, theoretical foundations of CSL (as described in chapter 14) are part of the didactic content of the course. A template is distributed to students that provides guidelines for CSL experiences. The four key components of CSL—planning, action, reflection, and celebration—are emphasized. This template is found in the appendices for chapter.

During the early semesters that these urban health electives were conducted, it became evident to faculty that many students needed guidance in the selection of a site in which to engage in their CSL experience. Faculty presented students with several options for venues where they might engage in CSL. It is important to note that these options included community sites where the wellness center has primary and secondary prevention programs already in place. In addition to providing a setting for the CSL activity, this strategy also provides students with awareness about the wellness center and the various public health initiatives that the center is engaged in with the community. Examples of possible CSL sites include schools, YMCAs, summer camp programs, and soup kitchens, as well as novel venues such as a racetrack. Students are not "assigned" to a specific community location; they self-select their CSL experience. Benefits of student self-selection include proximity to their dormitory or home and/or a CSL experience with a population that is of interest to the student (e.g., children, adolescents, seniors).

Because the students were traditional undergraduates and had class and clinical schedules during the week, finding CSL experiences to fit their schedules proved to be challenging. Several students expressed an interest in doing their CSL activity at the site of a weekend soup kitchen serving the homeless. The population at the soup kitchen was predominantly African American and was diverse in terms of age, including families with children, adults, and seniors.

After service at the soup kitchen, student reflections were profound. Some examples are the following:

- "I never knew there were so many families that needed to use a soup kitchen. I always thought that soup kitchens served only the elderly."
- "I now look at the homeless in a new way."

▧ "When I see a homeless person on the street, I now know that they have a story to tell."

In 2003, the lead faculty member for the course, who was also a full-time public health nurse at the wellness center, became aware of a mini-grant opportunity to support student CSL projects. The Pennsylvania Campus Compact Web site posted calls for applications for "Student Project Mini-Grant Proposals." Based upon previous students' positive experiences at the weekend soup kitchen, she wrote a proposal titled "Neat Feet" and was awarded a $500 mini-grant to support student activities at the site. The target population was the homeless population served by the weekend soup kitchen. All students enrolled in the course for three semesters (fall, spring, and summer of 2003) were made aware of this CSL project and had the option to select this site for their CSL experience.

There was a multilevel approach to the Neat Feet project. Early in the semester, a class seminar on the homeless population and their special needs was held. The public health nurse at the soup kitchen was the invited guest speaker. The dean and directors of the SONHS were also invited to attend the seminar. Mini-grant funds supported box lunches for all attendees. In-kind funding was provided by the SONHS for an honorarium for the guest speaker and space usage for the seminar. The following activities composed the "Neat Feet" project:

Appendix C.1

Activity	Person(s) Responsible	Due Date
Orient students to special foot care needs of the homeless	Faculty and nurse guest speaker who works at the site	By second week of course
Purchase foot care items (foot powder, athletic socks, gift bags)	Students	By mid-semester
Engage in foot soaks and foot inspections at the site	Students and staff at the site	By end semester
Provide recipients of foot care a gift bag with foot powder and new socks for their participation	Students	At time of CSL experience
Complete reflection documentation	Students	By end semester
Share reflections with classmates	Students	By end semester
Submit receipts for all items purchased to faculty	Students	By end semester
Submit receipts to university business office for student reimbursement	Faculty	At end of semester
Submit final report and copies of all receipts to funder	Faculty	By funder-specified due date

Four to six students participated in the Neat Feet initiative each semester. Student reflections post-CSL activity were overwhelmingly positive. Student reflections were done via various means, including short narratives, photographs with descriptions, artwork, and poetry. All reported the desire to continue the use of this setting for CSL experiences in the future. As of the writing of this book, four students are still actively engaged at this site on at least a quarterly basis.

LIFE Course: University of Delaware

Evelyn Hayes, PhD, APRN, BC

A personal health management and interdisciplinary university course, called the LIFE course, is an academic/community partnership. Building multidisciplinary outreach opportunities through academic/community partnerships was part of the learning experience for a group of 70 interdisciplinary students (nursing, health and exercise science, nutrition and dietetics) taking the course. Several community agencies (blood bank, Special Olympics, Lung Association of Delaware, Boys and Girls Clubs, Wellspring, American Cancer Society, Arthritis Association, food bank, Second Harvest, YMCA, and senior centers) were part of the partnership activity and had ongoing projects that students joined, while welcoming ideas from the students for new initiatives. The project was one of the "action lines" for several of the course concepts, such as time management, group membership and leadership, physical activity, and personal responsibility. It also underscored the concept of the positive impact of helping others with their health.

Groups of five to seven students developed and worked toward both individual and group goals and objectives and submitted final reports highlighting their accomplishments and providing personal reflections on their experience. Feedback from both students and community partnership agencies indicated that, although this group work was very time-consuming and challenging to coordinate, the experience was extremely beneficial personally and professionally. Coordination with the community partnership agencies also proved challenging for students. The outreach results and student learning, however, outweighed these obstacles. This project provided valuable learning for all of the students as they worked collaboratively toward common goals within their community. In addition, the project provided opportunities to students who had health career interests—opportunities not only to learn together, but also to share unique experiences related to their chosen profession. All of the students came away with a good sense of the objective of the course, the value of "Being a volunteer and making a difference in your community."

Asthma Safe Kids
In this outreach program, students partner with nurses to provide families of children with asthma with supplies and education about internal environmental triggers.

Nutrition Education to Elders
These CSL activities took place at a mental health day care facility, providing nutrition information for persons with mental health challenges.

Additional Student Service-Learning Activities

- Assisting at a senior community center with blood pressure screening, stroke screening, eating right classes (accompanied by cooking classes); and exercise classes (with discussion about the importance of exercise and recommendations on preventing osteoporosis).

- Senior students helping junior students in the skills lab, during both on- and off-hours.
- Administering flu shots at a flu clinic.
- Attending an Alzheimer's caregiver support group and teaching caregivers about the importance of and activities to promote stress relief for themselves.
- Participating in community health fairs, after-school programs, and summer camp programs.

Appendix

Chapter 5—NEEDS ASSESSMENT TOOL

_____ *SENIOR CENTER*   *07/2008*

The Nurses at the Center would like you to help us plan for future programs and activities that the Center could provide for you.

WE ARE ASKING YOU FOR SOME IDEAS FOR TOPICS FOR HEALTH PROMOTION AND WELLNESS THAT THE NURSE-MANAGED WELL-NESS CENTER COULD OFFER AT THE <u>SENIOR CENTER</u>.

- Please take some time to think about what ideas would be of interest to you.
- You can also bring this paper to the Center during office hours and talk to the nurse about what you are interested in the Center providing for the residents.

HERE ARE SOME IDEAS TO THINK ABOUT

Please √ check all topics that are interesting to you!

Health Promotion Topics:

_____ Diet-weight loss or weight gain
_____ Smoking, tobacco use—ways to stop
_____ Alcohol /Drug dependency
_____ Improving sleep (_____ snoring remedies)
_____ Exercise
_____ Ways to prevent illness/diseases
_____ Immunizations (for example, flu shots)
_____ Cancer Screening: (_____ Mammogram)(_____ Pap Smears)
  (_____ Bowels)(_____ Prostate)(_____ Skin)
_____ Vision Screening
_____ Blood Pressure monitoring
_____ Controlling stress incontinence (for example, leaking urine when you cough or sneeze)
_____ Screening for depression
_____ Preventing osteoporosis (for example, preventing bones from losing calcium and breaking easily)
_____ Testing your hearing
_____ Myths about aging
_____ Reminiscent Therapy (Sharing Your Memories)

Stress Management:

_____ Relaxation techniques   _____ Breathing exercises
_____ Positive self-talk   _____ Use of humor
_____ To learn about self-confidence _____ Management of retirement
_____ To learn about using our imagination to relax

How to Arrange and Organize Your Day-to-Day Activities and Living Space to Help You Get Around Better:

_____ For decreasing vision   _____ For loss of hearing

_____ For increasing forgetfulness   _____ For leaking urine

_____ For increasing unsteadiness on your feet

_____ For taking medication

_____ For anything else you can think of that wasn't mentioned

---

Managing Loss and Sorrow From Loss:

Safety

_____ Crime prevention   ____ Safe driving for older adults

_____ Life-saving alert devices   ____ Financial/material abuse or neglect

_____ Interpersonal violence, including sexual/physical pain or injury

_____ Accident prevention   ____ Psychological distress

(____ falls) (____ burns) (____ choking) (____ medication use)

(____ other, please list _____)

_____ Safety Assessments for visiting children

Legal Issues:

_____ Living wills/advanced directives   _____ Guardianship

_____ Durable power of attorney   _____ Other, please list

Age-Related Changes That May Occur:

_____ In the body; ____ In the mind; _____ Other, please list

_____

Information on Managing Specific Illnesses, Risk Factors, Diagnosis, Treatment, Self-Care: ____

Please list the illness/problems you are interested in learning about:

_____

_____

Extending Services to Family Members: ____

(Children, Grandchildren, Siblings, Friends) Please explain:

_____

_____

Please Add Any Comments or Ideas That You Would Like to Have Provided by the Wellness Center:

_____

_____

_____

_____

_____

_____

_____

_____
_____
_____
_____
_____
_____

Is There Anything Else You Would Like to Tell Us About the Wellness Center and the Services We Provide?

_____
_____
_____
_____
_____
_____
_____
_____
_____
_____
_____
_____

Thank you,
The Nurses at the _____ Wellness Center

Chapter 5—EXAMPLES OF STRATEGIC PLANS

Mission: The Mission of the _____ University School of Nursing Nurse-Managed Wellness Center (NMWC) is to provide wellness-oriented health care services to vulnerable populations. The goal is to deliver holistic and culturally competent care that promotes health, functioning and quality of life. The Center provides opportunities for interdisciplinary care experiences, service and research for students and faculty from the University. In all aspects of care, the uniqueness and strengths of the community and of each individual receiving care are maximized and respected. Confidentiality and awareness of each individual's rights to choose are maintained.

Vision: To be recognized as a world-wide model of an academic nurse-managed wellness center that adds to the body of knowledge that is nursing through service to students, faculty, clients, and community.

Broad Strategies

Education: Engage 100% of the undergraduate nursing students in clinical educational experiences in the Nurse-Managed Wellness Center (NMWC).

Scholarship: Involve students and faculty in interdisciplinary research projects and dissemination of research findings.

Service: Involve students, faculty, and volunteers in well-developed health and wellness programs and services.

Education: Expand the educational opportunities for undergraduate and graduate students through the Nurse-Managed Wellness Center (NMWC) to include care of vulnerable populations across the lifespan.

Goal Strategies:

- Collaborate with clinical coordinator to schedule students;
- Maintain and evaluate documentation system;
- Investigate opportunities for graduate research students;
- Update faculty/administration on a regular basis through total faculty meetings.

Scholarship: Assimilate the Boyer Model as a standard of scholarship through discovery, integration, and application of knowledge.

Goal Strategies:

- Continue leadership role in local, regional, and national organizations;
- Utilize School of Nursing and University resources effectively;
- Collaborate with author of the Omaha System;

- Develop a cyclical calendar for funding and timeline;
- Maintain program evaluation on an ongoing basis for students, faculty, and volunteers;
- Analyze and integrate the Retrospective Data Analysis Project;
- Participate in wellness manual–NNCC project.

Service: Develop evidenced-based service programming for vulnerable populations across the lifespan with input from academic and community stakeholders.

Goal Strategies:

- Investigate the Hartford Program;
- Investigate Board of Directors with more formal community representation;
- Expand faculty practice across the lifespan;
- Present updates to faculty/administration on a regular basis through total faculty meetings;
- Build relationships with City/County/State officials;
- Develop/evaluate/update Standard Operating Procedures.

_____ CENTER
EVALUATION PLAN 2007-2008

Problem

Homeless and indigent persons in _____ have difficulty accessing services for mental health, substance abuse, and medical care if they do not meet the criteria for Medicaid or Medicare or are unable to keep entitlements once they are secured.

Intervention

Create a facility where clients are served based on their perceived needs and not based on their ability to access funds for services

Goal

To provide state of the art services to disenfranchised clients at no cost that will enable them to more effectively deal with disorders and begin to access personal recovery

Objectives

1. Develop the infrastructure and staffing necessary to provide appropriate services to the identified population
2. Provide services at little or no cost to clients and when unable refer clients to other providers that will accept their care
3. Maintain high quality professionals as well as multidisciplinary students as part of the treatment teams
4. Identify and secure ongoing funding to sustain the activities of the clinic

Outcomes

1. Provide services to 300 un-reimbursable homeless and indigent clients each year in Cincinnati
2. Access the resources available for persons who have difficulty navigating current health care systems and document results
3. Stabilize funding for agency programs by increasing income by $100,000 in 2008
4. Track demographic data of program participants to demonstrate need
5. Advocate for the de-stigmatization of mental illness, addictions and poverty on all levels by writing letters, supporting legislation, and staying abreast of the political arena
6. Disseminate results and knowledge to stakeholders through presentations, research and publications

CENTER PROCESS EVALUATION

Process Objective 1: Develop the Infrastructure and Staffing Necessary to Provide Appropriate Services to the Identified Population

Performance Target	Data Source	Method for Data Collection	Person/s Responsible	Target Date to Accomplish	Status C or IP
1. Hire additional staff	Professional referrals	Interview	ED	Ongoing as needed	Completed
2. Reduce costs through ongoing evaluation of the budget	Financial reports and profit and loss statements	Current accounts	HRC Board and Financial Consultant	Summer 2007	In process
3. Complete CARF accreditation	CARF standards	Site visit scheduled Summer 2007	All staff	October 2007	In process
4. Complete ODADAS certification	ODADAS standards	Site visit	All staff	Completed February 2007	Completed
5. Collaborate with _____ around Medicaid reimbursement process	Consultation around Medicaid process	Personal interviews	ED and Directors	July 2007	Completed
6. Approach Mental Health Board for additional funds	Chair of _____. CFO and HRC personnel	Face to Face encounters	CEO and Financial Consultant	January 2008	In process

Process Objective 2: Provide Services at Little or No Cost to Clients and When Unable Refer Clients to Other Providers That Will Accept Their Care

Performance Target	Data Source	Method for Data Collection	Person/s Responsible	Target Date to Accomplish	Status C or IP
1. Continue to see a minimum of 50% un-reimbursable clients	Individual charts	Demographic studies	ED	Yearly reports	In process
2. Continue working with ongoing grantors	Current contracts	Personal collaboration	ED	At end of fiscal year	In process
3. Refer inappropriate clients out to other providers	Referral records on charts	Listing of appropriate referral agencies	Staff	Ongoing	In process
4. Evaluate the service delivery system and make appropriate changes	Staff meeting minutes and Team meeting minutes	Staff discussion with client recommendations	Staff	Ongoing	In process
5. Decrease costs by collaboration with like agencies	Financial reports and estimates of profit and loss	Personal collaboration	ED	July 2007	Completed

Process Objective 3: Maintain High Quality Professionals as Well as Multidisciplinary Students as Part of the Treatment Teams

Performance Target	Data Source	Method for Data Collection	Person/s Responsible	Target Date to Accomplish	Status C or IP
1. Provide a positive working environment for staff	Self evaluations	Evaluation forms	ED and appropriate directors	Ongoing	In process
2. Support staff through ongoing education and training	Personnel folders	Staff CEU records	Clinical directors	Ongoing with yearly training	In process
3. Complete yearly evaluations with staff	Personnel folders	Evaluation forms	ED and appropriate directors	Summer 2007	In process
4. Maintain academic connections to keep student flow constant	Personal connections to academic institutions	Contracts and letters of agreement	ED and Counseling faculty	Ongoing	In process
5. Mentor students within the multidisciplinary environment	Student folders and Team Meeting notes	Student supervisors	Senior staff	Ongoing	In process

Process Objective 4: Identify and Secure Ongoing Funding to Sustain the Activities of the Clinic

Performance Target	Data Source	Method for Data Collection	Person/s Responsible	Target Date to Accomplish	Status C or IP
1. Hire a grant writer	Personal referrals	Personal interview	ED	February 2007	Completed
2. Continue with fundraising activities	Development Committee Minutes	Number of fundraisers yearly	Development Committee	Ongoing	In process
3. Develop corporate partnerships	Liaison personnel from corporations	Number of contacts and visits	Board and ED	September 2007	Completed
4. Analyze data for program evaluation	Surveys, outcomes and demographic studies	Program statistics	ED	June of each year	Completed 2007
5. Publish article about the clinic	Literature and current practice and outcomes	Drafts of written work	ED with students and staff	Fall 2007	In process
6. Present data to stakeholders and professional organizations	Abstracts accepted and presentations completed four times in 2006-07	Program information and invitations	Academic faculty	Yearly	Completed 2007

_____ NURSING WELLNESS CENTER STRATEGIC PLAN

GOAL 1   Maintain Wellness Centers.

OBJECTIVES	STRATEGIES	RESPONSIBILITY	OUTCOMES	TIME	STATUS S/08
Maintain a task force to guide opera-tion of Nursing Wellness Center.	Task Force will consist of at least (1) representative from each level (sophomore, junior, senior and graduate).	Nursing Wellness Center Committee; Nursing Faculty	Management of Nursing Center will be a shared endeavor of faculty.	1 Year	
Assess satisfaction with care and service delivered.	Evaluate out-comes of client satisfaction through the use of surveys. Make program changes relevant to satisfaction outcomes.	Nursing Wellness Center Committee; Nursing Faculty	90% of clients will report sat-isfaction with service		Ongoing

GOAL 2

Promote Nursing Wellness Centers as an Integral Part of Educational Mission of the Department of Nursing.

OBJECTIVES	STRATEGIES	RESPONSIBILITY	OUTCOMES	TIME	STATUS S/08
Introduce students and faculty to the Nursing Wellness Center model of health care.	Provide information regarding clinic services to faculty and students.	Director Nursing Faculty	Participation in services offered will comprise 30% faculty and students		Ongoing
Provide clinical opportunities for graduate and undergraduate students.	Provide a summary of Nursing Wellness Center activities at faculty meetings. Encourage faculty/student participation in Nursing Wellness Center programs. Provide a supportive and collaborative environment for students. Develop and plan student clinical experiences at the Nursing Wellness Center. Precept and consult with students during clinical experiences related to the Nursing Wellness Center.	Director Nursing Wellness Center Committee; Nursing Faculty		5 years	Ongoing
Provide student access to a broad client base for special projects.	Implement special projects with faculty and students.	Faculty		5 years	Ongoing
Conduct formative and summative evaluations of student-directed health promotion services.	Devise student evaluation form to evaluate experiences with Nursing Wellness Center. Distribute student evaluation forms at the end of each semester. Analyze data from student evaluation form to evaluate student experience. Make program changes relevant to student input.	Nursing Wellness Center Committee Nursing Faculty		5 years	Ongoing

GOAL 3 — Provide Quality, Accessible, Affordable Health Promotion and Health Services to the Community.

OBJECTIVES	STRATEGIES	RESPONSIBILITY	OUTCOMES	TIME	STATUS S/08
Provide services to various populations in the community by exploring and responding to the health needs of the community.	Assess the health needs of various populations in the community. Market services to community members of all ages as potential clients.	Nursing Wellness Center Committee; Director Marketing/PR	Increase client number by 20% each year	1–5 years	Ongoing
Provide sound fiscal management to ensure sustainability.	Develop a business plan. Review and update business plan annually. Perform a cost-analysis of services and evaluate fee schedule annually. Seek new service contracts and agreements. Seek local, state, and federal funding to support identified needs and services. Maintain computerized client database.	Director Nursing Faculty	Maintain self-supporting status	1–3 years	Ongoing

GOAL 4 — Increase Community Awareness of Health Promotion and Health Care Practices Through Nursing Student/ Faculty-Directed Activities.

OBJECTIVES	STRATEGIES	RESPONSIBILITY	OUTCOMES	TIME	STATUS S/08
Meet with community leaders, alliances, organizations, and members to educate them about community-based services offered by nursing students and faculty of the Nursing Wellness Centers.	Communicate regularly with community groups and others regarding available services.	Director Nursing Faculty	Increase community involvement by 20%	2 years	Ongoing
Market student-directed and faculty-directed health promotion programs, screening, immunization projects through a variety of media.	Develop and utilize letterhead, brochure and logo to market Nursing Wellness Center. Market health promotion programs via radio, posters, flyers and Web announcements. Develop and maintain hospital/ university website. Send calendar of semester projects to affiliating agencies.	Director Nursing Faculty Marketing/PR	Increase community involvement and attendance by 20%	1-2 years	Ongoing

GOAL 5 — Provide Opportunities for Faculty Scholarship.

OBJECTIVES	STRATEGIES	RESPONSIBILITY	OUTCOMES	TIME	STATUS S/08
Provide opportunities for faculty scholarship.	Develop service contracts and agreements with community organizations to facilitate faculty practice interests. Establish incentives for faculty practice and/or opportunities to provide services at both the University and community levels. Facilitate faculty practice to enable ongoing certifications and specialization requirements.	Director Nursing Faculty	20% of faculty will be involved in practice via the Nursing Wellness Center	2-3 years	Ongoing
	Encourage collaborative research at Bloomsburg University and with partnering agencies/organizations. Disseminate information about past and current research studies conducted at the Nursing Wellness Center. Explore sources of funding for research at the Nursing Wellness Center. Update computer capabilities and databases to facilitate access, storage, and analysis of data.	Nursing Wellness Center Committee; Director Nursing Faculty		5 years	Ongoing

Chapter 5 — Policies and Procedures Table of Contents

I. MISSION, VISION AND GOAL STATEMENTS

II. POLICIES	Policy Number
Organizational Charts	001
Formulation and Review of Policies and Procedures	002
Official Documents of the Nurse-Managed Wellness Center	003
Confidentiality	004
Rights and Responsibilities of Clients	005
Client Satisfaction and Evaluation	006
Notification of Services	007
Eligibility to Receive Services from the NMWC	008
Client Consent	009
Clients' Right to Refuse Health Care Recommendations	010
Complaints and Grievances	011
Notification of Services to Health Care Providers	012
Health Record Access: Subpoenas and Court Orders	013
Disposal of Health Records	014
Personnel Identification and Use of Name Tags	015
Student and Faculty and Participants in the Center	016
Teaching Activities	017
Research Activities	018
Standard Precautions	019
Accessibility to Mobility Impaired Clients	020
Transportation of Clients To Nearest Hospital Emergency Department	021
Fire Safety	022
Smoking Regulations	023
Calibration of Sphygmomanometer	024
Material Safety Data Sheets	025
Omaha System	026
Reporting of Student Incident	027
Reporting of Student Health Incident	028
Policies for Additional Nurse-Managed Wellness Centers	029
Reports of Center Activities	030
Confidentiality of Client Health Records	031
Photocopying of Clients' Health Records	032

Continued

Chapter 5

Policies and Procedures Table of Contents (Cont'd)

Chapter 5 — JOB DESCRIPTIONS

JOB DESCRIPTION

Director, Nurse-Managed Wellness Centers (NMWC)

Responsibilities:

- Oversee the activities of the NMWC
- Carry out, update, evaluate, and revise the Policies and Procedures of the NMWC
- Oversee the functions of the staff of the NMWC
- Supervise the activities of the administrative assistant
- Administer grants, budgets
- Submit the formative and summative budget reports
- Oversee updates on the NMWC websites
- Schedule and chair meetings
- Develop job descriptions
- Hire and arrange to orient staff
- Oversee and maintain a safe environment and calibration records of updates of equipment
- Precept nursing students
- Coordinate interdisciplinary activities
- Coordinate, conduct research, program evaluation
- Responsible for QI activities
- Ensures and maintains confidentiality of all client records
- Participates in NMWC and National Nursing Center Consortium meetings and educational events
- Responsible for grant writing and seeking of ongoing funding

Required skills:

- Advanced Practice Nurse
- As per DUSON faculty requirements:
  - Licensed in PA
  - Malpractice insurance as per DUSON requirements
  - CPR certified
- Proficient in use of computer, online teaching

JOB DESCRIPTION

Manager, Nurse-Managed Wellness Center (NMWC)

Responsibilities:

- Assess, plan, implement and evaluate culturally competent client-centered care with a focus on wellness, disease prevention, and health promotion
- Perform functions of an advanced practice nurse as per the rules and regulations of Pennsylvania Board of Nursing
- Supervise nurse intern, clerical staff
- Schedule NMWC hours and activities
- Maintain safe work environment and calibration updates of equipment
- Responsible for maintaining, updating, policies of NMWC
- Precept nursing students
- Coordinate interdisciplinary activities
- Conduct research, program evaluation
- Responsible for QI activities at practice site
- Maintains documentation of activities at the NMWC
- Maintains confidentiality of all client records
- Participate in NMWC and National Nursing Center Consortium Meetings

Required skills:

- Advanced Practice Nurse
- As per DUSON clinical faculty requirements:
  - Licensed in PA
  - Malpractice insurance as per DUSON requirements
  - CPR certified
- Proficient in use of computer, online teaching

JOB DESCRIPTION

Registered Nurse

Overall Description:

Assess, plan, implement, and evaluate culturally competent client-centered care with a focus on wellness, health promotion, and disease prevention in the Nurse-Managed Wellness Center. Perform functions of a clinical nurse as per the rules and regulations set forth by the Pennsylvania State Board of Nursing.

Responsibilities:

- Carries out the Mission of the University and the Nurse-Managed Wellness Center NMWC;
- Implements philosophy and goals of the School of Nursing;
- Abides by all policies, procedures and guidelines of the NMWC;
- Maintains documentation and confidentiality of all client encounters and records;
- Plans, implements, evaluates, and maintains records on group-related educational related activities;
- Submits log books and documentation on client encounters/student participation/record of group encounters to NMWC office at least once a month;
- Schedules NMWC hours and activities;
- Precepts/acts as role model for student nurses;
- Assists with the collection of data for research, program evaluation, and quality improvement activities at site;
- Maintain a safe environment and calibration updates of equipment;
- Participate in NMWC meetings.

Required Skills:

- Registered Nurse
- As per DUSON faculty requirements:
  - ◆ Licensed in PA
  - ◆ Malpractice insurance as per DUSON requirements
  - ◆ CPR certified
- Proficient in use of computer, online teaching

JOB DESCRIPTION

Research Assistant

Nature of Work:
This position requires knowledge of the computer and the ability to initiate and complete literature searches. The research assistant reports directly to the Director of the NMWC.

Responsibilities:

- Perform data collection
- Assist with developing measure tools
- Assist with developing automated documentation system
- Assist with implementation and evaluation of automated documentation system
- Assist with developing record keeping to track projects, programs, and/or teaching materials
- Assists with writing of reports and scholarly papers
- Attends NMWC Meetings
- Assist at special events sponsored by the NMWC
- Assist with maintaining a safe and efficient work environment
- Other basic level nursing duties/computer related activities and assignments as necessary

Requirements:
Knowledge of databases, spreadsheets, and other programs to track data. This includes but is not limited to the following; good communication skills, considerable knowledge of spoken and written English, strong computer skills especially Microsoft Office Products, and ability to use email.

JOB DESCRIPTION

Administrative Assistant

Nature of work:

This position requires highly responsible clerical and technical skills. The Administrative Assistant will provide support to the NMWC team. Reports directly to the Director of the NMWC.

Illustrative Examples of Work:

Performs secretarial work and plans, organizes, and controls inventory. Orders all supplies, processes paper work for requisitions and purchases of NMWC related materials. Assists in planning and organizing social events related to NMWCs. Researches community agencies appropriate for referral/consultation.

General tasks:

Copying materials, entering data, ordering supplies, filing, assembling client charts, typing minutes of meetings, organizing files, and other clerical duties/computer related activities.

Skills Required:

The successful candidate will possess a minimum of an associate degree. Experience in working with diverse older adults a plus. Other skills include but are not limited to typing, knowledge of Microsoft Office Products, knowledge of arithmetic and simple financial record keeping, ability to use the computer, email, spreadsheets, knowledge of office equipment, practices and procedures, knowledge of laws, regulations, and policies governing operations of the NMWC. Ability to function efficiently and effectively during the planning and facilitation of special events, excellent telephone skills, and other community skills, ability to interact and work with other areas of the University.

THE _____ NURSING CENTER OF THE _____ UNIVERSITY SCHOOL OF NURSING

Job Title: Clinical Director

Minimum Qualifications:

- Current _____ State RN license
- Masters degree in Nursing
- 3 years Management or Administrative experience in a community–based health service and supervision of administrative and clinical staff

Primary Functions:

Uses the Center's Mission to ensure delivery of care that is client-centered, cost-effective, and evidence-based. Creates and maintains a positive teaching learning environment and coordinates the clinical and educational components of the Nursing Center with the School of Nursing

Position Description:

Coordinates the delivery of health services which includes:

Year One

- Establishment of clinic hours of function and system of client scheduling
- Supervision of care including:
  - ◆ Intake, triage, and center flow systems
  - ◆ Development of a health record recording system and maintenance
  - ◆ Development of a system of client follow-up
- Scheduling of faculty and student rotation through the center
- Collaboration with faculty and students in the development of health promotion, primary, secondary, and tertiary prevention programs and non-invasive nursing actions
- Creation of effective systems of communication among nursing center staff, faculty, and students and the wider Wellness Center staff and backup departments, e.g., IT
- Development of a fiscal oversight plan which includes:
  - ◆ Business plan development
  - ◆ Short and long-term objectives incorporating contracting, service delivery, network development, and credentialing of the Center
- Oversight of budget and preparation of monthly status report
- Development of a client information system that will provide demographic and other data to ensure:
  - ◆ Availability of data to funding sources, accrediting bodies, and faculty and students engaged in research projects
- Supervision and evaluation of support staff

- Establishment of a system of community outreach and a board of directors which includes, but is not limited to, catchment area leaders and Brooklyn Campus multidisciplinary representation
- Creation of a system of advertising and recruitment of clients
- Collaboration on grant writing

Year Two – In Addition to Year One:

- Establishment of a quality management program to ensure:
  - Development, implementation, and monitoring of policies, procedures, clinical protocols, and client outcomes
  - Compliance with nursing and nurse practitioner (NP) professional standards, accreditation and licensing criteria

Year Three – In Addition to Years One and Two:

- Establishment of system of graduate nursing faculty and NP student rotation for clinical practicum
- In collaboration with undergraduate and graduate faculty, establishment of a list of direct and primary care services to be provided to clients

Year Four – In Addition to Years One, Two, and Three:

- Evaluation of Center function and service for years one through three
- Establishment of goals for year five

Year Five – In Addition to Years One, Two, Three, and Four

- Written report re: Center performance over past five years
- Development of a strategic plan for next three years

Chapter 8 — Start-up Checklist

Checklist	Questions to Think About	Advice from Experts
Getting 501(c)3 Status	Will the center be an independent 501(c)3 or will it operate under the umbrella of another non-profit entity?	• Having its own 501c3 status allows a center greater financial freedom, but means greater scrutiny by the IRS. Information on the 501(c)3 filing process can be found at the IRS website http://www.irs.gov/charities/ index.html
Create an Governing or Advisory Board	What kind of skills do you need to start out? Who do you know who has these skills? What key community figures might be able to help?	• A board should be comprised of a group of dedicated people to share tasks, problem solve, and provide community input. In addition to community members, board members may be wellness center partners or people with expertise in fund raising, legal issues, and quality of care. • Find others in the community doing similar work and utilize them as resources.
Needs Assessment	Who in the community will be the target population? What is the population profile of the community? What is the status of the existing health care delivery system? What will be the range of services for the wellness center?	• Start with existing data such as the US Census, local health department, local United Way, or local hospital statistics to gain a better understanding of the needs of the community.
Resource Assessment	What services are other agencies in the area providing? Are there any gaps in services?	• This will help determine the type of services the center should offer and help identify potential partnerships and referral sources. • What are the resources available through the university or partnering agencies?
Mission Statement	What is the primary goal of the wellness center? What is the guiding principle behind starting the health center?	• The Mission helps guide decision-making and articulate the vision of the center to clients, staff, and funders. • Keep it short and clear. It should reflect the long-term vision for the center.
Space and Site Selection	Where should the wellness center be located to be most accessible to the target population? Are there licensing and zoning issues to be considered? How many rooms and offices are needed? Is a conference room needed? What hours of operation are needed?	• It is key to locate services in an area of need and to avoid duplication of existing services. • Take into consideration the number of clients to be served, how much space is needed for services—meetings, storage, and office space. • Is the space accessible to the handicapped and by public transportation?

Checklist	Questions to Think About	Advice from Experts
Laws and Regulations	What are the state, city, and local laws that pertain?	• Being well informed about rules and regulations will help prevent malpractice and other legal problems.
Licenses and Approvals	Is all the necessary paperwork completed to comply with relevant state and federal requirements? Is a laboratory needed? Will mental health services be provided and will a license be required for this service?	• A CLIA (Clinical Laboratory Improvements Amendments) certification is required for all blood testing. A CLIA waiver is needed for many screening tests performed in the community. CLIA "waived" tests. http://www.cms.hhs.gov/clia
Financial	How much money is needed to start the wellness center? Will services be provided for which fees can be charged? How and where will the center seek donations and grants?	• This will guide the services that will be provided by the wellness center and will help identify gaps.
Staffing	How many practitioners and support staff does the center need to operate? What credentials are required?	• Students and community volunteers can be excellent staffing resources for wellness centers. How can they be recruited and managed?
Insurance	What type of insurance will the center need? What type of liability coverage will the practitioners need?	• There are two types of liability coverage: professional liability insurance for the provider and comprehensive general liability policy for the facility. Requirements vary state-to-state. http://www.hpso.com • Can the wellness center be covered by the parent organization's insurance?
Quality Improvement/ Quality Assurance	How will the center measure the quality of services that the patients receive?	• A system must be in place to measure the quality of services provided and to evaluate the management of the wellness center. • The NNCC Quality Management Document is a helpful resource and is available on the NNCC website.

Adapted from Torrisi, D. L., & Hansen-Turton, T. (2005). Introduction in *Community and nurse-managed health centers: Getting them started and keeping them going.* New York: Springer Publishing Company.

Chapter 8—SAMPLE OF A CONTRACT WITH A LOCAL AGENCY

December 30, 200_

RE: Contractual Engagement for Specific Services Rendered by the Family Health Center of _____ to _____ on behalf of the National Nursing Centers Consortium in regards to the Lead Safe Babies Project, funded by the U.S. Environmental Protection Agency.

This Contract is to confirm our understanding for _____ as fiscal agent for the National Nursing Centers Consortium (hereinafter referred to as "NNCC") to engage Provider as an independent contractor to perform certain services for the NNCC under the terms and conditions set forth in this Letter of Agreement.

This letter, when signed by the director of the service provider and returned to the NNCC will constitute an agreement with the intention of being legally binding as follows:

1. Fiscal Agent hereby engages Provider as a consultant to provide Specific Services on behalf of the NNCC as stated in the attached Scope of Work.
2. The specific services the Provider will per form and the specific schedule for providing these services shall be in accordance with the provisions of Paragraph One (1) and may be as reasonably necessary or appropriate for the program to which it relates.
3. Provider shall perform all services under this Letter of Agreement in accordance with all applicable laws, regulations, other governing rule and standards, and the requirements of the program to which it relates, and shall perform all services in a manner consistent and in compliance with all accepted and prevailing standards for the proper performance of the same or similar services. The period of this contract shall be from September 1, 200_ to March 31, 200_; and may be terminated by either party with 3-day written notification to the other party, without cause or liability other than to compensate for services performed to the date of termination.
4. Subject to the availability of funds for this purpose, and in consideration of the specific services performed by Provider, and upon receipt of invoice and subsequent approval by Fiscal Agent under this Agreement, the NNCC shall pay a provider service fee of $__ up to 20 target clients, or 40 visits; this fee includes reimbursement for expenses incurred in the course of performing the above services. Work will be scheduled upon mutual agreement between the Provider and the NNCC.
5. Provider warrants that the performance will be of the highest professional quality.
6. Provider shall indemnify, defend and hold harmless the NNCC/Fiscal Agent from and against any and all losses, claims, actions, damages, liability, and expenses, including reasonable attorneys' fees incurred by the NNCC in connection with, arising out of, or resulting from any act or omission of Provider's agent, contractors, or servants pursuant to this contract.

7. NNCC/Fiscal Agent shall indemnify, defend and hold harmless Provider from and against any and all loses, claims, actions, damages, liability and expenses, including reasonable attorney's fees incurred by Provider in connection with or arising out of, or resulting from any act or omission of the NNCC's/Fiscal Agent's agents, contractors, employees, or servants pursuant to this contract.

8. The NNCC shall own all rights in and to the services provided, including copyrights and patents. Service Provider agrees to execute any documents that may be necessary to protect the NNCC's/Fiscal Agent's ownership rights.

9. Provider's relationship to the NNCC shall be one of independent contractor. Provider shall not in any number be deemed an agent or employee of the NNCC/ Fiscal Agent, and shall have no authority to bind or obligate, or incur any liability on behalf of the NNCC/Fiscal Agent, and no such authority shall be implied.

10. Pennsylvania law shall govern the validity, construction, interpretation, and effect of this Letter of Agreement.

11. Provider as an independent contractor, shall obtain and maintain during the term of the Letter of Agreement all required liability insurances to include, if applicable, professional malpractice liability insurance for the services provided under this Letter of Agreement and make every effort to name Fiscal Agent /NNCC as an additional insured under such policy.

Indicate your acceptance of the terms of the Letter of Agreement by signing in the space provided below. Please return a signed copy of this Letter of Agreement to Fiscal Agent. This Letter shall not be binding unless and until the PHMC receives a copy duly executed by you. Thank you.

_____

_____

Date

SCOPE OF WORK: LEAD SAFE BABIES PROVIDER
ENVIRONMENTAL PROTECTION AGENCY, REGION III NATIONAL NURSING CENTERS CONSORTIUM (NNCC)

Organizational Overview:
The National Nursing Centers Consortium (NNCC) was established in 1996, and is the only association of nurse-managed community health centers in the U.S. Currently, there are 40 NNCC-member nurse-managed health centers, all of which are located in or near medically underserved areas in both rural and urban communities.

Relationship of Provider to NNCC:
The Provider, an identified partner in the grant, is a member nurse-managed health center of the National Nursing Centers Consortium. In an effort to foster the growth and sustainability of the nursing centers, the NNCC contracts with its centers to perform outreach and education of the community. Stipends for reimbursement are based on time allocated to project and cost needs of the center.

Proposed Intervention:
Educational home and hospital visits to woman in their last trimester of pregnancy and mothers with newborn children up to 6 months of age.

Method/Target Areas:
Pregnant woman and new mothers that live in the rural Pennsylvania target area of Greene County. Referrals will be made by area nursing centers. Women can also refer themselves to the program, which will be advertised through posters and brochures.

Intervention/Statement of Work:
Outreach workers from the Provider will be responsible for the recruitment of clients from hospitals, community health centers, and clients of the nurse-managed health center. Referral/Intake information will be taken by staff at the nurse-managed health center and recorded in a program database. Upon receipt of the referral information, outreach workers will conduct introductory visits for up to 20 clients. Between 180 and 210 days later, a follow-up visit will be conducted; if the follow-up visit is not conducted within the designated timeframe, reimbursement will be lost. The visits will consist of in-house presentations and information on lead poisoning prevention techniques. Emphasis will be placed on actions the caregiver can use, such as hand washing, cleaning techniques and proper nutrition. A short pre-test will be administered to the caregiver to ascertain her level of knowledge about lead. Participants will be provided with incentives, including a "lead bucket" filled with supplies to enable them to clean the lead dust, e.g. sponges, detergent and hand soap. The healthcare worker will also teach the caregiver the appropriate way to avoid lead poisoning and present literature for the caregiver to keep. The follow-up visit will begin with the administration of a post-test, to measure retained knowledge about lead. During the visit, the outreach worker will review lead poisoning

prevention techniques discussed in the first visit. At the end of the visit, the outreach worker will present the caregiver with a gift card.

Target Audience:
Primary prevention geared toward pregnant women and new mothers living in the following target counties of rural Pennsylvania: Allegheny, Greene, Huntingdon, Montgomery, and Northumberland.

Time Period of Program: September 30, 200_ – March 31, 200_
During the grant period, the partners will meet regularly to review activities, report progress and problems, report client feedback, and correct problems. In order to ensure that the program meets its goals and objectives the NNCC will track the:

1. Number of lead education visits
2. Number of families lost to follow up
3. Increase in baseline knowledge, attitudes and behaviors regarding lead poisoning on the part of program clients
4. Lead levels of children screened.

Chapter 10—CHECKLIST FOR NUTRITIONAL HEALTH

DETERMINE YOUR NUTRITIONAL HEALTH

The Warning Signs of poor nutritional health are often overlooked. Use this Checklist to find out if you or someone you know is at nutritional risk.

Read the statements below. Circle the number in the "yes" column for those that apply to you or someone you know. For each "yes" answer, score the number in the box. Total your nutritional score.

• I have an illness or condition that made me change the kind and/or amount of food I eat.	2
• I eat fewer than 2 meals per day.	3
• I eat few fruits or vegetables or milk products.	2
• I have 3 or more drinks of beer, liquor or wine almost every day.	2
• I have tooth or mouth problems that make it hard for me to eat.	2
• I don't always have enough money to buy the food I need.	4
• I eat alone most of the time.	1
• I take 3 or more different prescribed or over-the-counter drugs every day.	1
• Without wanting to, I have lost or gained 10 pounds in the last 6 months.	2
• I am not always physically able to shop, cook and/or feed myself.	2
TOTAL	

Total Your Nutritional Score. If it's –

0-2 Good! Recheck your nutritional score in 6 months.

3-5 You are at moderate nutritional risk. See what can be done to improve your eating habits and lifestyle. Your office on aging, senior nutrition program, senior citizens center, or Health Department can help. Recheck your nutritional score in three months.

6 or more You are at high nutritional risk. Bring this Checklist the next time you see your doctor, dietitian, or other qualified health or social service professional. Talk with them about any problems you may have. Ask for help to improve your nutritional health.

Remember that Warning Signs suggest risk, but do not represent a diagnosis of any condition. Turn the page to learn more about the Warnings Signs of poor nutritional health.

These materials are developed and distributed by the Nutrition Screening Initiative, a project of:
AMERICAN ACADEMY OF FAMILY PHYSICIANS
THE AMERICAN DIETETIC ASSOCIATION
THE NATIONAL COUNCIL ON THE AGING, INC.
The Nutrition Screening Initiative • 1010 Wisconsin Avenue, NW • Suite 800 • Washington, DC 20007
The Nutrition Screening Initiative is funded in part by a grant from Ross Products Division of Abbott Laboratories, Inc.

Warnings Signs of Poor Nutritional Health

The Nutrition Checklist is based on the Warning Signs described below. Use the word DETERMINE to remind you of the Warning Signs.

Disease

Any disease, illness or chronic condition which causes you to change the way you eat, or makes it hard for you to eat, puts your nutritional health at risk. Four out of five older adults have chronic diseases that are affected by diet. Confusion or memory loss that keeps getting worse is estimated to affect one out of five or more of older adults. This can make it hard to remember what, when, or if you've eaten. Feeling sad or depressed, which happens to about one in eight older adults, can cause big changes in appetite, digestion, energy level, weight and well-being.

Eating Poorly

Eating too little and eating too much both lead to poor health. Eating the same foods day after day or not eating fruit, vegetables, and milk products daily will also cause poor nutritional health. One in five adults skip meals daily. Only 13% of adults eat the minimum amount of fruit and vegetables needed. One in four older adults drink too much alcohol. Many health problems become worse if you drink more than one or two alcoholic beverages per day.

Tooth Loss/Mouth Pain

A healthy mouth, teeth and gums are needed to eat. Missing, loose, or rotten teeth or dentures which don't fit well, or cause mouth sores, make it hard to eat.

Economic Hardship

As many as 40% of older Americans have incomes of less than $6,000 per year. Having less—or choosing to spend less—than $25-30 per week for food makes it very hard to get the foods you need to stay healthy.

Reduced Social Contact

One-third of all older people live alone. Being with people daily has a positive effect on morale, well-being, and eating.

Multiple Medicines

Many older Americans must take medicines for health problems. Almost half of older Americans take multiple medicines daily. Growing old may change the way we respond to drugs. The more medicines you take, the greater the chance for side effects such as increased or decreased appetite, change in taste, weakness, drowsiness, constipation, diarrhea, nausea, and others. Vitamins or minerals, when taken in large doses, act like drugs and can cause harm. Alert your doctor to everything you take.

Involuntary Weight Loss/Gain

Losing or gaining a lot of weight when you are not trying to do so is an important warning sign that must not be ignored. Being overweight or underweight also increases your chance of poor health.

Needs Assistance in Self Care
Although most older people are able to eat, one of every five have trouble walking, shopping, buying, and cooking food, especially as they get older.

Elder Years Above Age 80
Most older people lead full and productive lives. But as age increases, risk of frailty and health problems increase. Checking your nutritional health regularly makes good sense.

The Nutrition Screening Initiative • 1010 Wisconsin Avenue, NW • Suite 800 • Washington, DC 20007
The Nutrition Screening Initiative is funded in part by a grant from Ross Products Division of Abbott Laboratories, Inc.

Chapter 13—STUDENT HANDOUTS

Overview of Community Service and Learning

The following guidelines are adapted from: Greenberg, Jerrold (no date): *An Introduction to Service Learning in Health Education*. College Park, MD: University of Maryland Department of Health Education.

What is service and learning? Service and learning is a form of experiential learning in which students engage in activities that address both human and community needs coupled with structured learning environments. It is not the same as "internship" or "volunteerism." In these experiences, the beneficiary is the student. In service and learning, the direct beneficiary is the community group, or person/persons with whom the service and learning experience is conducted. The student benefits indirectly. The four phases of service and learning are described below.

Planning   Action   Refection   Celebration

1. *Planning:*   Preparing to engage in the activity. May include: needs assessment, interviews with key community members, site visits, etc.
2. *Action:*   Performing the service activity.
3. *Reflection:*   Drawing meaning from the activity. This may include journaling, writing a reflective paper, or group discussion.
4. *Celebration:*   Closing activity to reinforce future service. May include awards, certificates, or a closing meal.

Strategies for promoting reflection:

Orally: one-on-one meeting with instructor, group discussion, presentations

Writing: essays, poems, project reports, journals, writing a publishable article

Activities: dance movement, art, role play, gaming activities, scrapbooks, photo essays, poster display

The importance of leaving something behind: Service and learning participants should submit a product based on what was learned from the service activity. Products may include written comments, photographs, audiovisual materials, portfolios, or any other ways in which you can "leave something behind" for the organization you served and the group of students who take the course after you. Be creative!

Questions to reflect upon before during and after the service & learning experience:

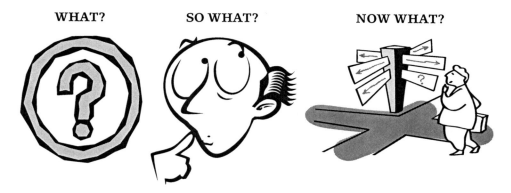

WHAT?   **SO WHAT?**   **NOW WHAT?**

What?

- What service did you perform?
- What people did you interact with?
- What was their role(s)?
- What career opportunities did you observe?

So What?

- What was the significance of the service?
- What did it mean to you personally?
- What are your positive and negative feelings about the service, the people you interacted with, and the overall experience?
- What skills, knowledge, theory learned in previous classroom settings did you apply?
- What skills/knowledge did you discover you lacked? How can you acquire these?

Now What?

- What impact did your service have on your everyday life?
- What impact might your service have on your lifelong learning?
- What insights did you gain that may help you during your career?
- What did this experience teach you about community involvement, citizenship, and your civic responsibility?

Sample Journal Reflection Questions

Reflect upon these reflective questions as you participate in your CSL experience. Answer the questions after you complete your CSL experience.

1. What was the most meaningful experience associated with your community service and learning activity?
2. What was your most frustrating experience and why? Could anything have been done to prevent your frustration?

3. How successful do you think you were in helping the people to whom you provided community service?
4. What new ways of looking at situations or people did you learn from this experience?
5. What ways of looking at situations or people do you think you have to improve upon?
6. Do you intend to continue to be involved in community service experiences? If not, why not? If yes, in what way(s) do you intend to continue to be involved?

MEM: 1/02 (rev. 12/04; 12/05; 7/08)

Chapter 14—HELPFUL TOOLS FOR FACULTY

Formulate questions that will help your students process their community-based work with regard to each of the following areas:

1. Course related texts, issues, and skills (Make this relevant to their course topic).
2. Existing mental models (of populations & tasks), unexamined cultural assumptions, untested values and priorities:
3. Contemporary issues and public policy-related questions (have students reflect on the given service learning project and examine how the student looks at it in a larger realm as it relates to public policy).

Adopted from Dr. Edward Zlotkowski 11/7/06 Workshop East Stroudsburg University

Example of a Community Service Learning Guide Used in an Undergraduate Psychiatric Mental Health Nursing Course
Community service learning is an opportunity to apply classroom knowledge in meeting the needs of the community. Service learning recognizes the reciprocal relationship between the university campus and those being served, thereby encouraging students to embrace their role as vested community members while assisting the community in seeing the promise in the students.

Students are required to complete a community service learning project to foster cultural awareness and competence, decrease stereotypes, and increase their skill and confidence in utilizing interpersonal skills with a vulnerable population. Culture is defined as a set of norms, values, and behaviors learned from membership in a group. Cultural competence is defined as acting on a set of values that leads one to seek knowledge about human differences and similarities, so that treat-nursing care can be delivered in a respectful and compassionate manner.

Students may volunteer at any agency that provided services to persons coping with mental disabilities, developmental disabilities, HIV/AIDS, domestic violence, homelessness, or Alzheimer's disease, or any other at-risk populations. Students meet with a contact person and develop objectives to accomplish in their ten hours of community service learning. Objectives should relate to the needs of both the students and the agency. An example of a student objective might be, "Student will understand what are the priority needs of a person who is homeless." An example of an agency objective may be, "Members of the group will demonstrate self-esteem by sharing a positive characteristic about themselves."

Requirements:

1. Prepare a 2-3 page APA paper responding to the following
   a. Describe the community service learning experience, including the agency, contact person, and participants, and the activity.
   b. Reflect what you learned as a result of your service learning experience. Share your feelings, ideas, and how you became more culturally competent. Share how your local/global understanding of community has grown and or changed.
   c. Incorporate a relevant article, preferably a research article.

Patty Hannon, PhD, RNc,
Associate Professor at East Stroudsburg University

Student Evaluation of the Community Service Learning Agency

Student Name _____ Date _____

Community Partner for Community Service Learning _____

Contact Person and Phone Number and/or email _____

Evaluation:

Would you recommend this Community Partner   Yes____ No____

Patty Hannon, Phd, RNc,
Associate Professor of East Stroudsburg University

Guidelines for Conducting Focus Groups

Size: 6 – 10 (12 maximum)

Duration: 1 – 1½ hrs.

Selection: Random (depending on objective, may include non-participants)

Facilitator: An interested party, but objective; someone not affected by results

Incentive: Offer incentives (i.e., give-aways, food)

Order:

Facilitator/Purpose Introduction

- who
- why group
- use of input
- appreciation of their time and input

Procedure

- "For the next hour and a half, I will facilitate a discussion among you that will help _____ to develop/improve/evaluate _____. As you can see, I will be tape recording our conversation. Also, _____ will be taking notes. You can be assured that all of your comments will be kept in strict confidence and that the report of the _____ will reflect collective response and will not list names of those who participated in this focus group."

Ground Rules

- "Just a couple of ground rules before we get started."
- "It is important that each of you is an active participant in the conversation. I will make every effort to allow each of you to speak. You do not need to raise your hand or be called on."
- "Only one person should speak at a time."
- "Try not to refer to your _____ (class, chapter, etc.) in your comments. You, of course, will use your own experience as a reference, but I would hope that you would try to represent other views as well."
- "Be honest in your remarks."

Script: Questions should be "scripted." Begin with "general" questions and progress to more specific questions.

Validity: Convening several different focus groups is preferable. After several groups, when the same answers are being relayed, one can conclude that the information is representative.

Adapted from: http://www.smu.edu/studentaffairs/files/Focus_Group_Guidelines.doc
This form was adapted from Form 5 (pages 343–352) of Martin, K., & Scheet, N. J. (1992). *The Omaha System: Applications for community health nursing.* Philadelphia: Saunders.

UNIVERSITY OF DELAWARE NURSING CENTER

OMAHA SYSTEM ASSESSMENT
ADMISSION/UPDATE

CLIENT NAME: _____

DATE: _____

CLIENT IDENTIFICATION NUMBER/CHART NUMBER:

_____

All data is Individual unless **NOTED** as Family.

PHYSIOLOGICAL DOMAIN

COGNITION

Adequate	Health Promotion	Potential	Impairment	Self Care	Low Priority

Other Provider _____

Oriented to:

Person ☐Y ☐N   Place ☐Y ☐N   Time ☐Y ☐N

Other Data/Risk Factors _____

_____

_____

_____

ROS   PE

_____ 01. Diminished judgment
_____ 02. Disoriented to time/place/person
_____ 03. Limited recall of recent events
_____ 04. Limited recall of long past events
_____ 05. Limited calculating/sequencing skills
_____ 06. Limited concentration
_____ 07. Limited reasoning/abstract thinking ability
_____ 08. Impulsiveness
_____ 09. Repetitive language/behavior
_____ 10. Other

CLIENT: K _____   B _____   S _____   FAMILY: K _____   B _____   S _____

SPEECH & LANGUAGE

Adequate	Health Promotion	Potential	Impairment	Self Care	Low Priority

Other Provider _____

Other Data/Risk Factors _____

_____

_____

_____

ROS   PE

_____ 01. Absent/abnormal ability to speak
_____ 02. Absent/abnormal ability to understand
_____ 03. Lacks alternative communication skills
_____ 04. Inappropriate sentence structure
_____ 05. Limited enunciation / clarity
_____ 06. Inappropriate work usage
_____ 07. Other

CLIENT: K _____   B _____   S _____   FAMILY: K _____   B _____   S _____

SENSORY-MOTOR FUNCTION

Adequate   Health Promotion   Potential   Impairment   Self Care   Low Priority

Other Provider _____

Pre-illness Level of Function

Indep. ☐   Assisted ☐   Dependent ☐

Describe: _____

_____

Current Mobility Status / Functional Limitations _____

_____

Activity Restrictions _____

_____

	ROS	PE
	_____	01. Limited range of motion
	_____	02. Decreased muscle strength
	_____	03. Decreased coordination
	_____	04. Decreased muscle tone
	_____	05. Increased muscle tone
	_____	06. Decreased sensation
	_____	07. Increased sensation
	_____	08. Decreased balance
	_____	09. Gait / ambulation disturbance
	_____	10. Difficulty managing activities of daily living
	_____	11. Tremor / seizures
	_____	12. Other

ADL Status:	I A D	IADL Status:	I A D		I A D	Assistive Devices
Bathe	☐ ☐ ☐	Telephone	☐ ☐ ☐	Preparing Meals	☐ ☐ ☐	☐ Cane ☐ Walker ☐ Wheelchair
Dress	☐ ☐ ☐	Traveling	☐ ☐ ☐	Housework	☐ ☐ ☐	☐ Raised Toilet Seat ☐ Commode
Toilet	☐ ☐ ☐	Shopping	☐ ☐ ☐	Medication	☐ ☐ ☐	☐ Shower chair/bench ☐ Hoyer
Transfer	☐ ☐ ☐	Money	☐ ☐ ☐			☐ Other _____
Feed	☐ ☐ ☐					

CLIENT: K _____   B _____   S _____   FAMILY: K _____   B _____   S _____

EYES/VISION

Adequate   Health Promotion   Potential   Impairment   Self Care   Low Priority

Other Provider _____

R _____   L _____   Correction _____

Other Data/Risk Factors _____

_____

_____

_____

	ROS	PE
	_____	01. Difficulty seeing small print/ calibration
	_____	02. Difficulty seeing distant objects
	_____	03. Difficulty seeing close objects
	_____	04. Absent/abnormal response
	_____	05. Abnormal results of vision screening
	_____	06. Squinting/blinking/tearing/blurring
	_____	07. Difficulty differentiating colors
	_____	08. Other

CLIENT: K _____   B _____   S _____   FAMILY: K _____   B _____   S _____

EARS/HEARING

Adequate   Health Promotion   Potential   Impairment   Self Care   Low Priority

Other Provider _____

R _____   L _____   Correction _____   ROS   PE

Other Data/Risk Factors _____

_____

_____

	ROS	PE
	_____	01. Difficulty hearing normal speech tones
	_____	02. Absent/abnormal response to sound
	_____	03. Abnormal results of hearing screening
	_____	04. Other

CLIENT: K _____   B _____   S _____   FAMILY: K _____   B _____   S _____

NOSE & SINUSES

Adequate   Health Promotion   Potential   Impairment   Self Care   Low Priority

Other Provider _____

ROS   PE

Other Data/Risk Factors _____

_____

_____

	ROS	PE
	_____	01. Frequent sinus infections
	_____	02. Blocked/painful sinuses
	_____	03. Difficulty determining smell
	_____	04. Rhinorrhea
	_____	05. Septal deviation
	_____	06. Other

CLIENT: K _____   B _____   S _____   FAMILY: K _____   B _____   S _____

MOUTH & THROAT

Adequate   Health Promotion   Potential   Impairment   Self Care   Low Priority

Other Provider _____

ROS   PE

Other Data/Risk Factors _____

_____

_____

	ROS	PE
	_____	01. Abnormalities of teeth
	_____	02. Sore/swollen/bleeding gums
	_____	03. Ill fitting dentures
	_____	04. Malocclusion
	_____	05. Other

CLIENT: K _____   B _____   S _____   FAMILY: K _____   B _____   S _____

RESPIRATION

Adequate   Health Promotion   Potential   Impairment   Self Care   Low Priority

Other Provider _____

	ROS	PE
Rate _____ Pattern _____	_____	01. Abnormal breath patterns
	_____	02. Unable to breathe independently
	_____	03. Cough
Lung Sounds _____	_____	04. Unable to cough/expectorate independently
	_____	05. Cyanosis
Other Data/Risk Factors _____	_____	06. Abnormal sputum
	_____	07. Noisy respirations
_____	_____	08. Rhinorrhea
	_____	09. Abnormal breath sounds
_____	_____	10. Other

CLIENT: K _____   B _____   S _____   FAMILY: K _____   B _____   S _____

CIRCULATION

Adequate   Health Promotion   Potential   Impairment   Self Care   Low Priority

Other Provider _____

Temp _____ AP (60 sec) _____ RP (60 sec) _____   ROS   PE

	ROS	PE
Rhythm/Quality Peripheral Pulses	_____	01. Edema
	_____	02. Cramping/pain of extremities
_____ _____	_____	03. Decreased pulses
	_____	04. Discoloration of skin/cyanosis
BP Sit Stand Lying	_____	05. Temperature change in affected area
R ____ L ____ R ____ L ____ R ____ L ____	_____	06. Varicosities
	_____	07. Syncopal episodes
	_____	08. Abnormal blood pressure reading
Edema _____	_____	09. Pulse deficit
	_____	10. Irregular heart rate
Other Data/Risk Factors _____	_____	11. Excessively rapid heart rate
	_____	12. Excessively slow heart rate
_____	_____	13. Anginal pain
	_____	14. Abnormal heart sounds/murmurs
_____	_____	15. Other

CLIENT: K _____   B _____   S _____   FAMILY: K _____   B _____   S _____

BREASTS

Adequate   Health Promotion   Potential   Impairment   Self Care   Low Priority

Other Provider _____

	ROS	PE
Other Data/Risk Factors _____	_____	01. Changes in size/shape
	_____	02. Abnormal discharge
_____	_____	03. Discoloration
	_____	04. Pain/tenderness
_____	_____	05. Other

CLIENT: K _____   B _____   S _____   FAMILY: K _____   B _____   S _____

NUTRITION

Adequate	Health Promotion	Potential	Impairment	Self Care	Low Priority

Other Provider _____

Ht _____ Wt _____ Diet _____

Other Data/Risk Factors _____

_____

_____

_____

_____

_____

ROS   PE

_____ 01. Weighs 10% more than average
_____ 02. Weighs 10% less than average
_____ 03. Lacks established standards for daily caloric/fluid intake
_____ 04. Exceeds established standards for daily caloric/fluid intake
_____ 05. Unbalanced diet
_____ 06. Improper feeding schedule for age
_____ 07. Non-adherence to prescribed diet
_____ 08. Unexplained/progressive weight loss
_____ 09. Hypoglycemia
_____ 10. Hyperglycemia
_____ 11. Other

CLIENT: K _____ B _____ S _____   FAMILY: K _____ B _____ S _____

DIGESTION/HYDRATION

Adequate	Health Promotion	Potential	Impairment	Self Care	Low Priority

Other Provider _____

Skin Turgor _____

_____

Other Data/Risk Factors _____

_____

_____

_____

_____

ROS   PE

_____ 01. Nausea/vomiting
_____ 02. Difficulty/inability to chew/swallow/digest
_____ 03. Indigestion
_____ 04. Reflux
_____ 05. Anorexia
_____ 06. Anemia
_____ 07. Ascites
_____ 08. Jaundice/liver enlargement
_____ 09. Decreased skin turgor
_____ 10. Cracked lips/dry mouth
_____ 11. Electrolyte imbalance
_____ 12. Other

CLIENT: K _____ B _____ S _____   FAMILY: K _____ B _____ S _____

BOWEL FUNCTION

Adequate   Health Promotion   Potential   Impairment   Self Care   Low Priority

Other Provider _____

Assistive Devices _____   ROS   PE

Other Data/Risk Factors _____

_____ 01. Abnormal frequency/consistency of stool
_____ 02. Painful defecation
_____ 03. Decreased bowel sounds
_____ 04. Blood in stools
_____ 05. Abnormal color
_____ 06. Cramping/abdominal discomfort
_____ 07. Incontinent of stool
_____ 08. Other

CLIENT: K _____   B _____   S _____   FAMILY: K _____   B _____   S _____

GENITO-URINARY FUNCTION

Adequate   Health Promotion   Potential   Impairment   Self Care   Low Priority

Other Provider _____

Ability to Void   ☐ Unassisted   ☐ Assisted   ROS   PE

_____ 01. Incontinent of urine

Catheter _____
_____ 02. Urgency/frequency
_____ 03. Burning/painful urination
_____ 04. Difficulty emptying bladder

Vaginal Discharge _____
_____ 05. Abnormal urinary frequency/amount
_____ 06. Hematuria

Other Data/Risk Factors _____
_____ 07. Abnormal discharge
_____ 08. Abnormal menstrual pattern
_____ 09. Abnormal lumps/swelling/ tenderness of male/female reproductive organs
_____ 10. Dyspareunia
_____ 11. Other

CLIENT: K _____   B _____   S _____   FAMILY: K _____   B _____   S _____

ORTHOPEDIC-MUSCULO-SKELETAL

Adequate   Health Promotion   Potential   Impairment   Self Care   Low Priority

Other Provider _____

Assistive Devices   ☐ Cane   ☐ Walker   ☐ Wheelchair   ROS   PE
     ☐ Raised Toilet Seat   ☐ Commode   _____ 01. Vertebrae abnormality
     ☐ Shower chair/bench   ☐ Hoyer   _____ 02. Pelvic girdle
     ☐ Commode   ☐ Splint/brace   _____ 03. LE abnormality
     ☐ Other _____   _____ 04. UE abnormality
     _____ 05. Phalangeal abnormality
     _____ 06. Other

Other Data/Risk Factors _____

CLIENT: K _____   B _____   S _____   FAMILY: K _____   B _____   S _____

PAIN

Health Promotion	Potential	Impairment	Self Care	Low Priority

Other Provider _____

Severity (0-10) _____ Location _____

Precipitating Factors _____

Controlled by _____

Other Data/Risk Factors _____

ROS PE
_____ 01. Expresses discomfort/pain
_____ 02. Elevated pulse/respirations/BP
_____ 03. Compensated movement/guarding
_____ 04. Restless behavior
_____ 05. Facial grimaces
_____ 06. Pallor/perspiration
_____ 07. Other

CLIENT: K _____   B _____   S _____   FAMILY: K _____   B _____   S _____

PRESCRIBED MEDICATION REGIMEN

Not Impairment	Adequate	Health Promotion	Potential	Self Care	Low Priority

Other Provider _____

Applicable

☐ Meds Reviewed   Meds in Home ☐Y ☐N

Plan to Obtain/Refill _____

Lacks knowledge of med:

☐ actions   ☐ dose   ☐ side effects

☐ adm/adm by _____

Other Data/Risk Factors _____

ROS PE
_____ 01. Deviates from prescribed dosage /
          schedule
_____ 02. Demonstrates side effects
_____ 03. Inadequate system for taking
          medication
_____ 04. Improper storage of medication
_____ 05. Fails to obtain refills appropriately
_____ 06. Fails to obtain immunization
_____ 07. Other

See care plan related to identified problem:

_____

CLIENT: K _____   B _____   S _____   FAMILY: K _____   B _____   S _____

INTEGUMENT

Adequate   Health Promotion   Potential   Impairment   Self Care   Low Priority

Other Provider _____

Braden Scale Risk Assessment Score: _____   ROS   PE

_____

Abnormalities (Describe/number if more than one)   _____ 01. Lesion
Location/Type: _____ 02. Rash
                                                         _____ 03. Excessively oily
_____   _____ 04. Excessively oily
                                                         _____ 05. Inflammation
Size (length, width, depth/stage, tunneling): _____ _____ 06. Pruritus
                                                         _____ 07. Drainage
                                                         _____ 08. Ecchymosis
_____   _____ 09. Hypertrophy of nails
                                                         _____ 10. Other
_____

Drainage (amount, type, odor):

_____

Tissue (color, granulation, necrosis):

_____

Signs/symptoms of infection: _____

_____

Other Data/Risk Factors _____

CLIENT: K _____   B _____   S _____   FAMILY: K _____   B _____   S _____

HAIR, SCALP & NAILS

Adequate   Health Promotion   Potential   Impairment   Self Care   Low Priority

Other Provider _____

                                                         ROS   PE
Other Data/Risk Factors _____   _____ 01. Changes in hair line/distribution
                                                         _____ 02. Excessively dry scalp
_____   _____ 03. Excessively oily scalp
                                                         _____ 04. Parasites
                                                         _____ 05. Changes in nails
_____   _____ 06. Other

CLIENT: K _____   B _____   S _____   FAMILY: K _____   B _____   S _____

PERSONAL HYGIENE

Not Assessed   Adequate   Health Promotion Potential   Impairment

Other Provider _____

	ROS	PE	
Assist of ☐ Self ☐ Other	_____	01. Inadequate laundering of clothing
	_____	02. Inadequate bathing
Other Data/Risk Factors _____	_____	03. Body odor
	_____	04. Inadequate shampooing/combing of hair
_____	_____	05. Inadequate brushing/flossing/ mouth care
_____	_____	06. Other

CLIENT: K _____   B _____   S _____   FAMILY: K _____   B _____   S _____

PHYSICAL ACTIVITY (In relation to present age/physical condition)

Not Assessed   Not Applicable   Adequate   Health Promotion   Potential   Impairment

	ROS	PE	
Other Data/Risk Factors _____	_____	01. Sedentary lifestyle
	_____	02. Inadequate/inconsistent exercise routine
_____	_____	03. Inappropriate type/amount of exercise for age/physical condition
_____	_____	04. Other

CLIENT: K _____   B _____   S _____   FAMILY: K _____   B _____   S _____

SLEEP & REST PATTERNS

Adequate   Health Promotion   Potential   Impairment

	ROS	PE	
	_____	01. Sleep/rest pattern disrupts family
	_____	02. Frequently wakes during night
Other Data/Risk Factors _____	_____	03. Somnambulism
	_____	04. Insomnia
_____	_____	05. Nightmares
_____	_____	06. Insufficient sleep/rest for age/ physical condition
	_____	07. Other

CLIENT: K _____   B _____   S _____   FAMILY: K _____   B _____   S _____

INTERPERSONAL RELATIONSHIP

Not Assessed   Not Applicable   Adequate   Health Promotion   Potential   Impairment

                     ROS   PE

_____ 01. Difficulty establishing/maintaining relationships

_____ 02. Minimal shared activities

_____ 03. Incongruent values/goals

Other Data/Risk Factors _____ _____ 04. Inadequate interpersonal communication skills

_____ _____ 05. Prolonged, unrelieved tension

_____ 06. Inappropriate suspicion/ manipulation/ compulsion

_____ _____ 07. Other

CLIENT: K _____   B _____   S _____   FAMILY: K _____   B _____   S _____

SOCIAL CONTACT

Not Assessed   Adequate   Health Promotion   Potential   Impairment

Support System: _____ ROS   PE

_____ 01. Limited social contact

Other Data/Risk Factors _____ _____ 02. Uses health care provider for social contact

_____ _____ 03. Minimal outside stimulation/ leisure time activities

_____ _____ 04. Other

CLIENT: K _____   B _____   S _____   FAMILY: K _____   B _____   S _____

EMOTIONAL STABILITY

Not Assessed   Not Applicable   Adequate   Health Promotion   Potential   Impairment

                     ROS   PE

_____ 01. Sadness/hopelessness/ worthlessness

Other Data/Risk Factors _____ _____ 02. Apprehension/undefined fear

_____ 03. Loss of interest/involvement in activities/self-care

_____ _____ 04. Narrowed perceptual focus

_____ 05. Scattering of attention

_____ _____ 06. Flat affect

_____ 07. Irritable/agitated

_____ _____ 08. Purposeless activity

_____ 09. Difficulty managing stress

_____ _____ 10. Somatic complaints/chronic suicide

_____ 11. Expresses wish to die/attempts suicide

_____ 12. Other

CLIENT: K _____   B _____   S _____   FAMILY: K _____   B _____   S _____

SPIRITUAL DISTRESS

Not Assessed   Not Applicable   Adequate   Health Promotion   Potential   Actual

    ROS   PE

Church/Minister: _____   _____ 01. Expresses spiritual concerns

_____ 02. Disrupted spiritual rituals

Funeral Home: _____   _____ 03. Disrupted spiritual trust

_____ 04. Conflicting spiritual beliefs and medical regimen

Other Data/Risk Factors _____   _____ 05. Other

_____

CLIENT: K _____   B _____   S _____   FAMILY: K _____   B _____   S _____

GRIEF

Not Assessed   Not Applicable   Adequate   Health Promotion   Potential   Impairment

    ROS   PE

Other Data/Risk Factors _____   _____ 01. Fails to recognize normal grief responses

_____   _____ 02. Difficulty coping with grief responses

_____   _____ 03. Difficulty expressing grief responses

_____   _____ 04. Conflicting stages of grief process among family/individuals

_____   _____ 05. Other

CLIENT: K _____   B _____   S _____   FAMILY: K _____   B _____   S _____

HUMAN SEXUALITY

Not Assessed   Not Applicable   Adequate   Health Promotion   Potential   Impairment

    ROS   PE

Other Data/Risk Factors _____   _____ 01. Difficulty recognizing consequences of sexual behavior

_____   _____ 02. Difficulty expressing intimacy

_____   _____ 03. Sexual identity confusion

_____ 04. Sexual value confusion

_____   _____ 05. Dissatisfied with sexual relationships

_____   _____ 06. Other

CLIENT: K _____   B _____   S _____   FAMILY: K _____   B _____   S _____

ROLE CHANGE

Not Assessed   Not Applicable   Adequate   Health Promotion   Potential   Impairment

                                                  ROS   PE

Other Data/Risk Factors _____ _____ 01. Involuntary reversal of traditional
male/female roles

_____ _____ 02. Involuntary reversal of dependent/
independent roles

_____ _____ 03. Assumes new role

_____ _____ 04. Loses previous role

_____ _____ 05. Other

CLIENT: K _____   B _____   S _____   FAMILY: K _____   B _____   S _____

CARETAKING/PARENTING

Adequate   Health Promotion   Potential   Impairment   Self Care   Low Priority

                                          Other Provider _____

Primary Caregiver _____ ROS   PE

_____ 01. Difficulty providing physical care /
safety

Caregiver able and willing to provide care   ☐ Yes ☐ No   _____ 02. Difficulty providing emotional
nurturance

_____ 03. Difficulty providing cognitive learning
experiences and activities

Other Data/Risk Factors _____ _____ 04. Difficulty providing preventive and
therapeutic health care

_____ _____ 05. Expectations incongruent with stage
of growth and development

_____ _____ 06. Dissatisfaction / difficulty with
responsibilities

_____ _____ 07. Neglectful

_____ 08. Abusive

_____ 09. Other

CLIENT: K _____   B _____   S _____   FAMILY: K _____   B _____   S _____

NEGLECTED ADULT

Not Assessed   Not Applicable   Health Promotion   Potential   Actual

	ROS	PE	Actual
Other Data/Risk Factors _____	_____		01. Lacks adequate physical care
	_____		02. Lacks emotional nurturance/support
	_____		03. Lacks appropriate stimulation / cognitive experiences
_____	_____		04. Inappropriately left alone
_____	_____		05. Lacks necessary supervision
	_____		06. Inadequate / delayed medical care
_____		_____	07. Other

CLIENT: K _____   B _____   S _____   FAMILY: K _____   B _____   S _____

ABUSED ADULT

Not Assessed   Not Applicable   Health Promotion   Potential   Actual

	ROS	PE	Actual
	_____		01. Harsh / excessive discipline
	_____		02. Welts / bruises / burns
Other Data/Risk Factors _____	_____		03. Questionable explanation of injury
	_____		04. Attacked verbally
_____	_____		05. Fearful / hypervigilant behavior
	_____		06. Violent environment
_____	_____		07. Consistent negative messages
	_____		08. Assaulted sexually
_____	_____		09. Other

CLIENT: K _____   B _____   S _____   FAMILY: K _____   B _____   S _____

FAMILY PLANNING

Not Assessed   Not Applicable   Adequate   Health Promotion   Potential   Impairment

	ROS	PE	
Other Data/Risk Factors _____	_____		01. Inappropriate / insufficient knowledge of family planning
	_____		02. Inaccurate / inconsistent use of family planning methods
_____	_____		03. Dissatisfied with present family planning method
_____	_____		04. Other

CLIENT: K _____   B _____   S _____   FAMILY: K _____   B _____   S _____

GROWTH & DEVELOPMENT OF ADULT

Not Assessed   Not Applicable   Adequate   Health Promotion   Potential   Impairment

	ROS	PE	
	_____		01. Age-inappropriate behavior
Other Data/Risk Factors _____	_____		02. Inadequate achievement / maintenance of developmental tasks
_____	_____		03. Other

CLIENT: K _____   B _____   S _____   FAMILY: K _____   B _____   S _____

ENVIRONMENTAL DOMAIN

INCOME

Not Assessed	Not Applicable	Adequate	Health Promotion	Potential	Impairment

ROS   PE

_____ 01. Low / no income

Source _____ _____ 02. Uninsured medical expenses

Other Data/Risk Factors _____ _____ 03. Inadequate money management

_____ 04. Able to buy necessities only

_____ 05. Difficulty buying necessities

_____ _____ 06. Other

CLIENT: K _____   B _____   S _____   FAMILY: K _____   B _____   S _____

SANITATION

Adequate	Health Promotion	Potential	Deficit	Self Care	Low Priority

Other Provider _____

*Other _____ ROS   PE

_____ 01. Soiled living area

_____ 02. Inadequate food storage / disposal

Other Data/Risk Factors _____ _____ 03. Insects / rodents

_____ 04. Foul odor

_____ 05. Inadequate water supply

_____ _____ 06. Inadequate sewage disposal

_____ 07. Inadequate laundry facilities

_____ _____ 08. Allergens

_____ 09. Infectious / contaminating agents

_____ _____ 10. Other

CLIENT: K _____   B _____   S _____   FAMILY: K _____   B _____   S _____

RESIDENCE

Adequate	Health Promotion	Potential	Deficit	Self Care	Low Priority

Other Provider _____

Description of safety measures required to protect client from injury:

ROS   PE

_____ 01. Structurally unsound

_____ 02. Inadequate heating / cooling

_____ 03. Steep stairs

_____ 04. Inadequate / obstructed exits / entries

_____ _____ 05. Cluttered living space

_____ _____ 06. Unsafe storage of dangerous objects / substances

Other Data/Risk Factors _____ _____ 07. Unsafe mats / throw rugs

_____ 08. Inadequate safety devices

_____ _____ 09. Presence of lead based paint

_____ 10. Unsafe gas / electrical appliances

_____ _____ 11. Inadequate / crowded living space

_____ 12. Homeless

_____ _____ 13. Other

CLIENT: K _____   B _____   S _____   FAMILY: K _____   B _____   S _____

NEIGHBORHOOD / WORKPLACE SAFETY

Not Assessed   Adequate   Health Promotion   Potential   Deficit

ROS   PE

Other Data/Risk Factors _____   _____ 01. High crime rate
_____ 02. High pollution level
_____ 03. Uncontrolled animals
_____   _____ 04. Physical hazards
_____ 05. Unsafe play area
_____   _____ 06. Other

CLIENT: K _____   B _____   S _____   FAMILY: K _____   B _____   S _____

COMMUNICATION WITH COMMUNITY RESOURCES

Adequate   Health Promotion   Potential   Impairment   Self Care   Low Priority

Other Provider _____

Food Resources _____   ROS   PE

_____ 01. Unfamiliar with options / procedures
for obtaining services
_____   _____ 02. Difficulty understanding roles /
regulations of service providers
_____   _____ 03. Unable to communicate concerns to
service providers
Transportation Resources _____   _____ 04. Dissatisfaction with services
Other Data/Risk Factors _____   _____ 05. Language barrier
_____ 06. Inadequate / unavailable resources
_____   _____ 07. Other

CLIENT: K _____   B _____   S _____   FAMILY: K _____   B _____   S _____

HEALTH CARE SUPERVISION

Adequate   Health Promotion   Potential   Impairment

ROS   PE

_____ 01. Fails to obtain routine medical /
dental evaluation
Other Data/Risk Factors _____   _____ 02. Fails to seek care for symptoms
requiring medical / dental evaluation
_____ 03. Fails to return as requested to
_____   physician / dentist
_____ 04. Inability to coordinate multiple
_____   appointments / regimens
_____ 05. Inconsistent source of medical /
_____   dental care
_____ 06. Inadequate prescribed medical /
_____   dental regimen
_____   _____ 07. Other

CLIENT: K _____   B _____   S _____   FAMILY: K _____   B _____   S _____

SUBSTANCE USE

Not Assessed   Not Applicable   Adequate   Health Promotion   Potential   Impairment

                                                 ROS   PE

Other Data/Risk Factors _____   _____ 01. Abuses over-the-counter / street
                                                                    drugs
_____   _____ 02. Abuses alcohol
                                                            _____ 03. Smokes
_____   _____ 04. Difficulty performing normal routines
                                                            _____ 05. Reflex disturbances
_____   _____ 06. Behavior change
                                                            _____ 07. Other

CLIENT: K _____   B _____   S _____   FAMILY: K _____   B _____   S _____

TECHNICAL PROCEDURE

Not Applicable   Adequate   Health Promotion   Potential   Impairment   Self   Low
                                                                                             Care   Priority

                                                                    Other Provider _____

                                                            ROS   PE

Procedure(s) _____   _____ 01. Unable to demonstrate / relate
                                                                    procedure accurately
_____   _____ 02. Does not follow / demonstrate prin-
                                                                    ciples of safe / aseptic techniques
                                                            _____ 03. Procedure requires nursing skill
Supplies in Home ☐ Yes ☐ No   Plan to Obtain _____   _____ 04. Unable / unwilling to perform proce-
                                                                    dures without assistance
_____   _____ 05. Unable / unwilling to operate special
                                                                    equipment
Other Data/Risk Factors _____   _____ 06. Other person(s) unable / unavailable
                                                                    to assist
_____   _____ 07. Other

CLIENT: K _____   B _____   S _____   FAMILY: K _____   B _____   S _____

Promoting Healthy Lifestyles in Delaware Project

BP/Stroke Risk Screening

DEMOGRAPHICS (circle all that apply)

ID # _____ Date: _____ Gender: M — F

Race:

1—White   2—Black   3—American Indian/Eskimo/Aleut

4—Asian/Pacific Islander   5—other   6—unknown

Ethnicity:

1—Hispanic origin   2—Non-Hispanic origin   3—unknown

Marital Status:

1—single   2—married   3—separated

4—divorced   5—domestic partner   6—widowed

7—common law partner   8—other   9—unknown

Primary Language Spoken:

1—English   2—Spanish   3—other

Employment Status:

1—full-time   2—part-time

3—unemployed/seeking work   4—unemployed not seeking work

5—retired   6—student

7—disabled   8—other

9—unknown

Household Size: _____ (enter numeric value)

Highest Grade Completed:

1—no education   2—less than 8th grade

3—some high school   4—GED high school equivalency diploma

5—high school graduate   6—some technical or trade school

8—some college   7—technical or trade school graduate

9—college graduate   10—any post-graduate work

11—unknown

Citizenship Status:

1—US citizen   2—not a US citizen   3—Unknown

Usual Source of Health Care:

1—nursing center   2—other physician/nurse

3—city district health center   4—community health center

5—emergency room   6—none

7—unknown

Heart Rate: _____

Rhythm: (circle one) Regular / Irregular

BP:_____ (circle one) sitting / standing / lying

Edema: _____

Other Data/Risk Factors: _____

_____

CIRCULATION

Modifiers: (select one)

Adequate   Health Promotion   Potential   Impairment

Signs/Symptoms of Impairment: (select those that apply)

1—edema	2—cramping
3—decreased pulses	4—discoloration of skin/cyanosis
5—temperature change in affected area	6—varicosities
7—syncopal episodes	8—abnormal BP
9—pulse deficit	10—irregular heart rate
11—excessively rapid heart rate	12—excessively slow heart rate
13—anginal pain	14—abnormal heart sounds/murmurs
15—other	

Problem Rating Scale for Outcomes: (rate from 1 to 5)

Knowledge _____   Behavior_____   Status_____

PRESCRIBED MEDICATION REGIMEN

Modifiers: (select one)

Adequate   Not Applicable   Health Promotion   Potential

Meds Reviewed: ❒ Yes ❒ No   **Meds in Home:** ❒ Yes ❒ No

Plan to Obtain/Refill _____

Lacks Knowledge of Med:

❒ actions   ❒ dose   ❒ side effects   ❒ adm./adm.by:_____

Signs/Symptoms of Impairment: (select those that apply)

1—deviates from prescribed dosage/schedule	4—improper storage of medication
2—demonstrates side-effects	5—unable/unwilling to perform procedure
3—inadequate system for taking medication	6—fails to obtain immunization
	7—other

Problem Rating Scale for Outcomes: (rate from 1 to 5)

Knowledge _____   Behavior_____   Status_____

RESPIRATION

Modifiers: (select one)

Adequate   Health Promotion   Potential   Impairment

Rate: _____ **Pattern:** _____

Lung sounds: _____

Other Data/Risk Factors: _____

_____

Signs/Symptoms of Impairment: (circle all that apply)

1—abnormal breath patterns   2—unable to breathe independently
3—cough   4—unable to cough/expectorate independently
5—cyanosis   7—noisy respirations
6—abnormal sputum   9—abnormal breath sounds
8—rhinorrhea
10—other

Problem Rating Scale for Outcomes: (rate from 1 to 5)
Knowledge _____   **Behavior** _____   **Status** _____

COMMUNICATION WITH COMMUNITY RESOURCES

Modifiers: (select one)

Adequate   Health Promotion   Potential   Impairment

Food Resources: _____

Transportation Resources: _____

Other Data/Risk Factors: _____

_____

Signs/Symptoms of Impairment: (circle all that apply)

1—unfamiliar with options/procedures   2—difficulty understanding roles/
   or obtaining services   regulations of service providers
3—unable to communicate concerns   4—dissatisfaction with services
   to service providers   5—language barrier
6—inadequate/unavailable resources   7—other

Problem Rating Scale for Outcomes: (rate from 1 to 5)
Knowledge _____   **Behavior** _____   **Status** _____

Problem Classification Scheme (Circle all that apply)

Domain I: Environmental
1. Income
2. Sanitation
3. Residence
4. Neighborhood/workplace safety
5. Other

Domain II: Psychosocial
6. Communication with community resources
7. Social contact
8. Role change
9. Interpersonal relationship
10. Spiritual distress
11. Grief
12. Emotional stability
13. Human sexuality
14. Care taking/parenting
15. Neglected child/adult
16. Abused child/adult
17. Growth and development
18. Other

Sources: **SF-12 Health Status Questionnaire +Martin, K. & Scheet, N.J. (1992). *The Omaha System: Applications for Community health nursing.* Philadelphia: Saunders.

Domain III: Physiological
19. Hearing
20. Vision
21. Speech and language
22. Dentition
23. Cognition
24. Pain
25. Consciousness
26. Integument
27. Neuro-musculo-skeletal function
28. Respiration
29. Circulation
30. Digestion-hydration
31. Bowel function
32. Genito-urinary function
33. Antepartum/postpartum
34. Other

Domain IV: Health Related Behaviors
35. Nutrition
36. Sleep and rest patterns
37. Physical activity
38. Personal hygiene
39. Substance misuse
40. Family planning
41. Health care supervision
42. Prescribed medication regimen
43. Technical procedure
44. Other

Problem Rating Scale for Outcomes:

Knowledge: The ability of the client to remember and interpret information

1	2	3	4	5
No knowledge	Minimal knowledge	Basic knowledge	Adequate knowledge	Superior knowledge

Behavior: The observable responses, actions, or activities of the client fitting the occasion or purpose

1	2	3	4	5
Not appropriate	Rarely appropriate	Inconsistently appropriate	Usually appropriate	Consistently appropriate

Status: The condition of the client in relation to objective and subjective defining characteristics

1	2	3	4	5
Extreme Signs/Symptoms	Severe Signs/Symptoms	Moderate Signs/Symptoms	Minimal Signs/Symptoms	No Signs/Symptoms

DEMOGRAPHICS (circle all that apply)

ID # _____ Date: _____ Gender: M — F

Race:

1—White   2—Black   3—American Indian/Eskimo/Aleut

4—Asian/Pacific Islander   5—other   6—unknown

Ethnicity:

1—Hispanic origin   2—Non-Hispanic origin   3—unknown

Marital Status:

1—single   2—married   3—separated

4—divorced   5—domestic partner   6—widowed

7—common law partner   8—other   9—unknown

Primary Language Spoken:

1—English   2—Spanish   3—other

Employment Status:

1—full-time   2—part-time

3—unemployed/seeking work   4—unemployed not seeking work

5—retired   6—student

7—disabled   8—other

9—unknown

Household Size: _____ (enter numeric value)

Highest Grade Completed:

1—no education   2—less than 8th grade

3—some high school   4—GED high school equivalency diploma

5—high school graduate   6—some technical or trade school

8—some college   7—technical or trade school graduate

9—college graduate   10—any post-graduate work

11—unknown

Citizenship Status:

1—US citizen   2—not a US citizen   3—Unknown

Usual Source of Health Care:

1—nursing center   2—other physician/nurse

3—city district health center   4—community health center

5—emergency room   6—none

7—unknown

Height_____ Weight _____ BMI _____

NUTRITIONAL SCREENING TOOL

Read the statements below. Circle the number in the yes column for those that apply to you or someone you know. For each yes answer, score the number in the box. Total your score.

	YES
I have an illness or condition that made me change the kind and/or amount of food I eat.	2
I eat fewer than 2 meals per day.	3
I eat few fruits or vegetables or milk products.	2
I have 3 or more drinks of beer, liquor or wine almost every day.	2
I have tooth or mouth problems that make it hard for me to eat.	2
I don't always have enough money to buy the food I need.	4
I eat alone most of the time.	1
I take 3 or more different prescribed or over-the-counter drugs a day.	1
Without wanting to, I have lost or gained 10 pounds in the last 6 months.	2
I am not always physically able to shop, cook and/or feed myself.	2
TOTAL	

Scoring: 0-2—No problem;   3-5—Moderate risk;   6+ High risk

Diet History:

Breakfast_____

Lunch _____

_____

Dinner _____

_____

_____

Snacks _____

NUTRITION

Modifiers: (select one)

Adequate   Health Promotion   Potential   Impairment

Signs/Symptoms of Impairment: (select those that apply)

1—weighs 10 percent <u>more than</u> average

2—weighs 10 percent <u>less than</u> average

3—<u>lacks</u> established standards for daily caloric/fluid intake

4—<u>exceeds</u> established standards for daily caloric/fluid intake

5—unbalanced diet

6—improper feeding schedule for age

7—nonadherence to prescribed diet

8—unexplained/progressive weight loss

9—hypoglycemia

10—hyperglycemia

11—other

Problem Rating Scale for Outcomes: (rate from 1 to 5)

Knowledge _____   **Behavior**_____   **Status**_____

COMMUNICATION WITH COMMUNITY RESOURCES

Modifiers: (select one)

Adequate   Health Promotion   Potential   Impairment

Food Resources:_____

Transportation Resources: _____

Other Data/Risk Factors: _____

_____

Signs/Symptoms of Impairment: (circle all that apply)

1—unfamiliar with options/procedures or obtaining services

2—difficulty understanding roles/ regulations of service providers

3—unable to communicate concerns to service providers

4—dissatisfaction with services

5—language barrier

6—inadequate/unavailable resources

7—other

Problem Rating Scale for Outcomes: (rate from 1 to 5)

Knowledge _____   **Behavior**_____   **Status**_____

Omaha System Format: Problem Classification Scheme (Circle all that apply)

Domain I: Environmental
1. Income
2. Sanitation
3. Residence
4. Neighborhood/workplace safety
5. Other

Domain II: Psychosocial
6. Communication with community resources
7. Social contact
8. Role change
9. Interpersonal relationship
10. Spiritual distress
11. Grief
12. Emotional stability
13. Human sexuality
14. Care taking/parenting
15. Neglected child/adult
16. Abused child/adult
17. Growth and development
18. Other

Sources: SF-12 Health Status Questionnaire. Martin, K. & Scheet, N.J. (1992). *The Omaha System: Applications for Community health nursing.* Philadelphia: Saunders. Lipschitz: (1992). Am Fam Physician.

Domain III: Physiological
19. Hearing
20. Vision
21. Speech and language
22. Dentition
23. Cognition
24. Pain
25. Consciousness
26. Integument
27. Neuro-musculo-skeletal function
28. Respiration
29. Circulation
30. Digestion-hydration
31. Bowel function
32. Genito-urinary function
33. Antepartum/postpartum
34. Other

Domain IV: Health Related Behaviors
35. Nutrition
36. Sleep and rest patterns
37. Physical activity
38. Personal hygiene
39. Substance misuse
40. Family planning
41. Health care supervision
42. Prescribed medication regimen
43. Technical procedure
44. Other

Problem Rating Scale for Outcomes:

Knowledge: The ability of the client to remember and interpret information

1	2	3	4	5
No knowledge	Minimal knowledge	Basic knowledge	Adequate knowledge	Superior knowledge

Behavior: The observable responses, actions, or activities of the client fitting the occasion or purpose

1	2	3	4	5
Not appropriate	Rarely appropriate	Inconsistently appropriate	Usually appropriate	Consistently appropriate

Status: The condition of the client in relation to objective and subjective defining characteristics

1	2	3	4	5
Extreme Signs/Symptoms	Severe Signs/Symptoms	Moderate Signs/Symptoms	Minimal Signs/Symptoms	No Signs/Symptoms

Promoting Healthy Lifestyles in Delaware Project

General Health Inventory

DEMOGRAPHICS (circle all that apply)

ID # _____ Date: _____ Gender: M — F

Race:

1—White   2—Black   3—American Indian/Eskimo/Aleut
4—Asian/Pacific Islander   5—other   6—unknown

Ethnicity:

1—Hispanic origin   2—Non-Hispanic origin   3—unknown

Marital Status:

1—single   2—married   3—separated
4—divorced   5—domestic partner   6—widowed
7—common law partner   8—other   9—unknown

Primary Language Spoken:

1—English   2—Spanish   3—other

Employment Status:

1—full-time   2—part-time
3—unemployed/seeking work   4—unemployed not seeking work
5—retired   6—student
7—disabled   8—other
9—unknown

Household Size: _____ (enter numeric value)

Highest Grade Completed:

1—no education   2—less than 8th grade
3—some high school   4—GED high school equivalency diploma
5—high school graduate   6—some technical or trade school
8—some college   7—technical or trade school graduate
9—college graduate   10—any post-graduate work
11—unknown

Citizenship Status:

1—US citizen   2—not a US citizen   3—Unknown

Usual Source of Health Care:

1—nursing center   2—other physician/nurse
3—city district health center   4—community health center
5—emergency room   6—none
7—unknown

Heart Rate: _____ **Rhythm:** (circle one) Regular / Irregular

BP:_____ (circle one) sitting / standing / lying

Edema: _____

Other Data/Risk Factors: _____

SF-12 HEALTH STATUS QUESTIONNAIRE

Please answer the following questions as accurately and honestly as possible. Your responses will help us serve you better.

1. In general, would you say your health is: (Circle one)

Excellent   **Very Good**   **Good**   **Fair**   **Poor**

The following items are about activities you might do during a typical day. Does your health limit you in these activities? If so, how much?

	Yes, limited a lot	Yes, limited a little	No, not limited at all
2. Moderate activities, such as moving a table, pushing a vacuum cleaner, bowling, or playing golf.	❏	❏	❏
3. Climbing several flights of stairs a day.	❏	❏	❏

During the *past 4 weeks*, have you had any of the following problems with your work or other regular daily activities as a *result of your physical health?*

	Yes	No
4. Accomplished less than you would like	❏	❏
5. Were limited in the kind of work or other activities	❏	❏

During the *past 4 weeks*, have you had any of the following problems with your work or other regular daily activities as a *result of any emotional problems* such as feeling depressed or anxious?

	Yes	No
6. Accomplished less than you would like	❏	❏
7. Didn't do work or other activities as carefully as usual	❏	❏

8. During the *past 4 weeks*, how much did pain interfere with your normal work (including both work outside the home and housework)?

   Not at all   A little bit   Moderately   Quite a bit   Extremely

These questions are about how you feel and how things have been with you during the past 4 weeks. For each question, please give the one answer that comes closest to the way you have been feeling.

	All of the time	Most of the time	A good bit of the time	Some of the time	A little of the time	None of the time
9. Have you felt calm and peaceful?	❏	❏	❏	❏	❏	❏
10. Did you have a lot of energy?	❏	❏	❏	❏	❏	❏
11. Have you felt downhearted and blue?	❏	❏	❏	❏	❏	❏
12. During the *past 4 weeks*, how much of the time has your physical health or emotional health problems interfered with your social activities (like visiting friends, relatives, etc.)?	❏	❏	❏	❏	❏	❏

SOCIAL CONTACT

Modifiers: (select one)

Adequate   Health Promotion   Potential   Impairment

Support System:_____

Other Data/Risk Factors: _____

Signs/Symptoms of Impairment: (select those that apply)

1—limited social contact   2—uses health care provider for social contact

3—minimal outside stimulation/leisure time activities   4—other

Problem Rating Scale for Outcomes: (rate from 1 to 5)

Knowledge _____   Behavior_____   Status_____

PHYSICAL ACTIVITY

Modifiers: (select one)

Adequate   Not assessed   Not applicable   Health Promotion   Potential

Data/Risk Factors:_____

Signs/Symptoms of Impairment: (select those that apply)

1—sedentary life style   2—inadequate/inconsistent exercise routine

4—other   3—inappropriate type/amount of exercise for age/
                                          physical condition

Problem Rating Scale for Outcomes: (rate from 1 to 5)

Knowledge _____   Behavior_____   Status_____

EMOTIONAL STABILITY

Modifiers: (select one)

Adequate   Not assessed   Not capable   Health Promotion   Potential

Data/Risk Factors:_____

Signs/Symptoms of Impairment: (select those that apply)

1—sadness/hopelessness/worthlessness   2—apprehension/undefined fear

3—loss of interest/involvement in   4—narrowed perceptual focus
   activities/self-care   5—scattering of attention

6—flat affect   7—irritable/agitated

8—purposeless activity   9—difficulty managing stress

10—somatic complaints/chronic fatigue   11—expresses wish to die/
                                                                            attempts suicide
12—other

Problem Rating Scale for Outcomes: (rate from 1 to 5)

Knowledge _____   Behavior_____   Status_____

Problem Classification Scheme (Circle all that apply)

Domain I: Environmental
1. Income
2. Sanitation
3. Residence
4. Neighborhood/workplace safety
5. Other

Domain II: Psychosocial
6. Communication with community resources
7. Social contact
8. Role change
9. Interpersonal relationship
10. Spiritual distress
11. Grief
12. Emotional stability
13. Human sexuality
14. Care taking/parenting
15. Neglected child/adult
16. Abused child/adult
17. Growth and development
18. Other

Sources: **SF-12 Health Status Questionnaire +Martin, K. & Scheet, N.J. (1992). *The Omaha System: Applications for community health nursing.* Philadelphia: Saunders.

Domain III: Physiological
19. Hearing
20. Vision
21. Speech and language
22. Dentition
23. Cognition
24. Pain
25. Consciousness
26. Integument
27. Neuro-musculo-skeletal function
28. Respiration
29. Circulation
30. Digestion-hydration
31. Bowel function
32. Genito-urinary function
33. Antepartum/postpartum
34. Other

Domain IV: Health Related Behaviors
35. Nutrition
36. Sleep and rest patterns
37. Physical activity
38. Personal hygiene
39. Substance misuse
40. Family planning
41. Health care supervision
42. Prescribed medication regimen
43. Technical procedure
44. Other

Problem Rating Scale for Outcomes:

Knowledge: The ability of the client to remember and interpret information

1	2	3	4	5
No knowledge	Minimal knowledge	Basic knowledge	Adequate knowledge	Superior knowledge

Behavior: The observable responses, actions, or activities of the client fitting the occasion or purpose

1	2	3	4	5
Not appropriate	Rarely appropriate	Inconsistently appropriate	Usually appropriate	Consistently appropriate

Status: The condition of the client in relation to objective and subjective defining characteristics

1	2	3	4	5
Extreme Signs/Symptoms	Severe Signs/Symptoms	Moderate Signs/Symptoms	Minimal Signs/Symptoms	No Signs/Symptoms

Omaha System Information Sheet
Collection of Additional Problems/Needs Not Captured on Survey Form

Client Identification:

Problems/Needs: Circle ALL that apply.   (Scale 1-5)   Target #

Environmental Domain	Modifier: Circle	K	B	S	HT	SU	CM	TP
1. Income	Imp - Pot - H. Prom							
2. Residence	Imp - Pot - H. Prom							
3. Sanitation	Imp - Pot - H. Prom							
4. Neighborhood/Workplace Safety	Imp - Pot - H. Prom							
5. Other	Imp - Pot - H. Prom							
Psychosocial Domain	**Modifier: Circle**	**K**	**B**	**S**	**HT**	**SU**	**CM**	**TP**
6. Communication with Community Resources	Imp - Pot - H. Prom							
7. Social Contact	Imp - Pot - H. Prom							
8. Role Change	Imp - Pot - H. Prom							
9. Interpersonal Relationship	Imp - Pot - H. Prom							
10. Spiritual Distress	Imp - Pot - H. Prom							
11. Grief	Imp - Pot - H. Prom							
12. Emotional Stability	Imp - Pot - H. Prom							
13. Human Sexuality	Imp - Pot - H. Prom							
14. Caretaking/Parenting	Imp - Pot - H. Prom							
15. Neglected Child/Adult	Imp - Pot - H. Prom							
16. Abused Child/Adult	Imp - Pot - H. Prom							
17. Growth/Development	Imp - Pot - H. Prom							
18. Other	Imp - Pot - H. Prom							
Physiological Domain	**Modifier: Circle**	**K**	**B**	**S**	**HT**	**SU**	**CM**	**TP**
19. Hearing	Imp - Pot - H. Prom							
20. Vision	Imp - Pot - H. Prom							
21. Speech & Language	Imp - Pot - H. Prom							
22. Dentition	Imp - Pot - H. Prom							
23. Cognition	Imp - Pot - H. Prom							
24. Pain	Imp - Pot - H. Prom							
25. Consciousness	Imp - Pot - H. Prom							
26. Integument	Imp - Pot - H. Prom							
27. Neuro-musculoskeletal	Imp - Pot - H. Prom							
28. Respiration	Imp - Pot - H. Prom							
29. Circulation	Imp - Pot - H. Prom							
30. Digestion-hydration	Imp - Pot - H. Prom							
31. Bowel Function	Imp - Pot - H. Prom							
32. Genito-urinary	Imp - Pot - H. Prom							
33. Ante-/post-partum	Imp - Pot - H. Prom							
34. Other	Imp - Pot - H. Prom							
Health-Rel Beh Domain	**Modifier: Circle**	**K**	**B**	**S**	**HT**	**SU**	**CM**	**TP**
35. Nutrition	Imp - Pot - H. Prom							
36. Sleep and Rest Patterns	Imp - Pot - H. Prom							
37. Physical Activity	Imp - Pot - H. Prom							
38. Personal Hygiene	Imp - Pot - H. Prom							
39. Substance Use	Imp - Pot - H. Prom							
40. Family Planning	Imp - Pot - H. Prom							
41. Health Care Supervision	Imp - Pot - H. Prom							
42. Prescribed Medication Regimen	Imp - Pot - H. Prom							
43. Technical Procedure	Imp - Pot - H. Prom							
44. Other	Imp - Pot - H. Prom							

Intervention (Rx) Categories

1. Anatomy/physiology
2. Behavior modification
3. Bladder care
4. Bonding
5. Bowel care
6. Bronchial hygiene
7. Cardiac care
8. Caretaking/parenting skills
9. Cast care
10. Communication
11. Coping skills
12. Day care/respite
13. Discipline
14. Dressing change/wound care
15. Durable medical equipment
16. Education
17. Employment
18. Environment
19. Exercises
20. Family planning
21. Feeding procedures
22. Finances
23. Food
24. Gait training
25. Growth/development
26. Homemaking
27. Housing
28. Interaction
29. Lab findings
30. Legal system
31. Medical/dental care
32. Med action/side effects
33. Med administration
34. Med set-up
35. Mobility/exercise
36. Nursing care, supplementary
37. Nutrition
38. Nutritionist
39. Ostomy care
40. Other community resources
41. Personal care
42. Positioning
43. Rehabilitation
44. Relaxation/breathing techniques
45. Rest/sleep
46. Safety
47. Screening
48. Sickness/injury care
49. Signs/sxs—mental/emotional
50. Signs/sxs—physical
51. Skin care
52. Social work/counseling
53. Specimen collection
54. Spiritual care
55. Stimulation/nurturance
56. Stress management
57. Substance use
58. Supplies
59. Support group
60. Support system
61. Transportation
62. Wellness
63. Other

Key
Imp = impairment
Pot = potential impairment
H. Prom = health promotion
K = Knowledge
B = Behavior
S = Status
HT = health teaching
SU = surveillance
CM = case management
TP = technical procedure

Source: Martin, K. & Scheet, N.J. (1992). The Omaha System: Applications for community health nursing. Phila: Saunders

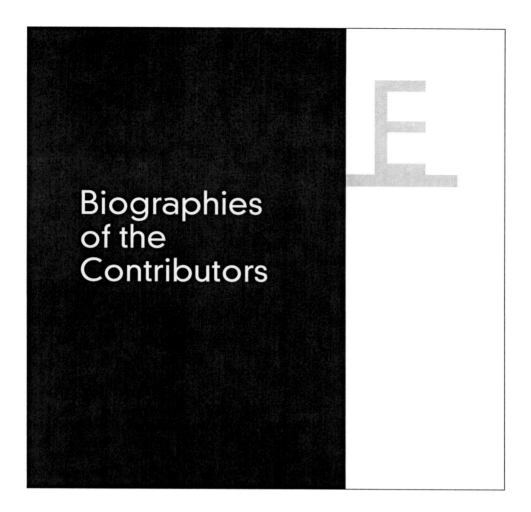

Julie Cousler Emig, MSW, LSW

Ms. Julie Cousler Emig is the vice president of health promotion and wellness at Congreso de Latinos Unidos, where she has served Philadelphia's Latino community for a decade. With a master's degree in social work from Temple University, she is a licensed social worker with a historical commitment to women's health and family wellness. She is the architect and principal investigator of a federally funded clinical research project serving the community's most vulnerable teen parents. She daily speaks publicly to the unique needs of Latinos on numerous local and state boards and committees related to domestic violence, behavioral health, HIV/AIDS, and family health. Ms. Cousler Emig is also a member of the board of directors of the Women's Medical Fund, where she has held various positions, including chair of the board. She is a new director to the Seybert Foundation's board of directors, and she is active in her Northern Liberties neighborhood, where she is working to preserve valuable green space for the community.

Diane M. Haleem, PhD, RN

Dr. Diane Haleem is an associate professor at Marywood University, teaching in both the undergraduate bachelor of science in nursing program and the graduate nursing administration program. She earned both her PhD and bachelor of science (nursing) from Boston College, and received her master's degree in nursing administration at University of California, Los Angeles, and a certificate in special studies in administration and management from Harvard University. She is past director of the Nursing Wellness Project. Her research work and interests are harm reduction and college drinking, parents' influence associated with their sons and daughters drinking, Service Learning (students learning while giving back to the community), NCLEX Success (strategies that work), and Good Work (students reflecting on themes associated with good work, which include reflecting on what good work is, beliefs and values, goals, responsibilities, and excellence).

Evelyn (Lyn) R. Hayes, PhD, MPH, FNP-BC

Dr. Evelyn Hayes received her bachelor of science in nursing from Cornell University, New York Hospital School of Nursing; an MPH in public health nursing from the University of North Carolina School of Public Health (Chapel Hill); and a PhD in higher education from Boston College. In addition, she completed a post-master's certificate as family nurse practitioner at the University of Massachusetts at Amherst and is a certified family nurse-practitioner. She has valuable practice experience in acute care institutions and in the community. Currently, she is a professor in the School of Nursing, College of Health Sciences, at the University of Delaware. In this role, she has had teaching responsibilities at both the undergraduate and graduate levels and experience with distance learning. She also serves as director of the UD Nursing Center and co-coordinator of nurse-practitioner program. Dr. Hayes has consulted with faculty in Taiwan and Panama.

Dr. Hayes and her nursing center colleagues have been awarded multiple competitive grants to promote care for the underserved and education of students. A strong advocate of health promotion, Dr. Hayes served as project director and co-investigator of a U.S. Public Health Service grant promoting healthy lifestyles in Delaware. The "Picture Yourself a Nurse Campaign" was also launched. Dr. Hayes completed the NNCC Beck Fellowship Program and served on the Education and Research Committee of NNCC. She has governor appointments to state committees and councils, including the Council on Aging and Adults with Physical Disabilities, and leadership positions in professional and community organizations. Dr. Hayes gives many presentations at national and international professional meetings and has published in multiple journals.

Caroline Helton, MS, MN, RN

Ms. Caroline Helton is an instructor in the Department of Nursing at Missouri State University. She received her BSN from Central Missouri State University, Warrensburg, MO; a master of teacher education degree from Pittsburg State

University, Pittsburg, KS; and a master of nursing degree from University of Kansas. Her research interests include delivery of health care to vulnerable populations; students' perceptions and beliefs about poverty; and teaching strategies to engage student learning, such as service learning, student-to-student peer mentoring, and simulations. Professor Helton teaches in the undergraduate generic BSN and BSN completion programs. She is also program director for the generic BSN program and serves on the graduate faculty.

Susan M. Hinck, PhD, RN

Dr. Susan Hinck is a Robert Wood Johnson Health Policy Fellow in Washington, DC, and formerly was an associate professor at Missouri State University Department of Nursing. Her clinical and research background is in gerontology, rural health, and cultural issues, with experience in rehabilitation, home health care, and administration. She has a BSN from Central Missouri University, MN from the University of Kansas, and PhD in nursing from Saint Louis University. She completed a postdoctoral fellowship with the John A. Hartford Center for Nursing Excellence at Oregon Health and Science University in 2004 and was honored as a 2006 Hartford Institute Geriatric Nursing Research Scholar at New York University.

Kathryn L. Hope, PhD, RN

Dr. Kathryn Hope is an associate professor and head of the Department of Nursing, which includes nursing and public health programs, at Missouri State University in Springfield, Missouri. Dr. Hope received her BSN from Washburn University of Topeka, an MA in nursing from the University of Iowa in child health and nursing education, a PhD in nursing from the University of Kansas, and a post-master's certificate as a family nurse-practitioner from the University of Missouri-Columbia. Dr. Hope has had a long interest in health care of underserved populations, especially children. Her research interests focus on the health of the underserved and at-risk populations.

Penny Killian, MSN, RN, MHPNP

Ms. Penny Killian is an assistant professor with Drexel University, College of Nursing and Health Professions. She teaches community/public health nursing, nurses building a healthy community, and global health policy and issues in the undergraduate BSN nursing program, as well as ethics in the graduate nursing program. Ms. Killian received her bachelor's degree from Jersey City State College in New Jersey and her master's degree from LaSalle University in Pennsylvania. She is a clinical specialist in public health nursing and has recently completed a post-master's degree from the Medical College of Pennsylvania and Hahnemann University. She has been certified as a psychiatric nurse-practitioner in the state of Pennsylvania. She attended the Alden Bioethics Institute and received a certificate in clinical bioethics.

Ms. Killian has long worked with her community, serving on the Board of Health in South Brunswick Township, NJ, as Chairman and Vice Chairman; with the chronically mentally ill in Middlesex County, NJ; and as a consultant evaluating community health, health care education, and program needs. Her special interests are health promotion, disease prevention in a community setting, and the provision of psychiatric and primary care services to the persistently mentally ill living in community settings. Ms. Killian is currently working with the public health nursing team of Drexel College of Nursing and Health Profession in the 11th Street Corridor and in the larger Philadelphia communities with community members, church groups, and local schools, and with community health nursing students, to deliver health-promotion and disease-prevention programs. She and a Drexel University colleague have been engaged in community research related to depression in African American women and exploration of the health issues of selected immigrant/refugee populations. An important part of this community work has been collaboration and linkage with many Philadelphia government and nongovernmental agencies that support mental health and overall wellness.

Eunice S. King, PhD, RN

Dr. Eunice King is senior program officer and director of research and evaluation for the Independence Foundation in Philadelphia, where she manages grant making and projects related to the nurse-managed health center funding initiative and conducts evaluations of other Foundation projects. A nurse for almost 40 years, Dr. King graduated from the Johns Hopkins Hospital School of Nursing in 1968, received her BSN from the University of Pennsylvania in 1971, received a master's degree in psychiatric mental health nursing from Boston University in 1973, and received a PhD in human development from Bryn Mawr College in 1988. Her professional experience has included nine years as a psychiatric nursing clinical specialist in a variety of health care settings, teaching in baccalaureate and master's programs in nursing, and research. Upon completion of her doctoral studies, she joined the research faculty of the Fox Chase Cancer Center, where, for the next nine years, she conducted behavioral research in mammography utilization and smoking cessation, was the recipient of NCI funding, and coauthored numerous publications. Prior to joining the Independence Foundation in 2000, she was associate dean for research for three years in the MCP Hahnemann School of Nursing in Philadelphia.

Since joining the Independence Foundation in 2000, Dr. King has led and consulted with grantees on a number of data-related projects. From 2001 through 2004, she worked with the NNCC and eight Philadelphia-area nurse-managed centers to select and implement an electronic practice management and medical record system, which was funded by the Independence Foundation. In addition, she has provided consultation to the Community College of Philadelphia on the development of the health-promotion data-collection tool and continues to participate in the NNCC's data committee meetings. Her experience as a researcher, combined with her working knowledge of nurse-managed health centers and related health policy issues, has given her a broad perspective on the data needed from nurse-managed centers, as well as on the process for collecting valid, high-quality data.

Maureen E. Leonardo, MN, CRNP, CNE, FNP-BC

Ms. Maureen Leonardo is an associate professor in the School of Nursing at Duquesne University in Pittsburgh, Pennsylvania, as well as a nurse practitioner for Western Pennsylvania Family Medical Associates in Jeannette, Pennsylvania. She is a certified nurse educator and has spent the last 20 years in academia, planning and implementing educational programs. In addition, as a certified family nurse practitioner, she has an active practice and considerable experience working with older adults. In the last 12 years, she has focused on health and wellness activities with the older adult.

Ms. Leonardo received a bachelor of science in nursing degree from Indiana University of Pennsylvania and an MSN as a clinical nurse specialist from the University of Pittsburgh. She earned a post-master's certificate as a family nurse practitioner from Duquesne University. She is a member of the National Organization of Nurse Practitioner Faculties, National League for Nursing, and Sigma Theta Tau International (Epsilon Phi Chapter), as well as the National Nursing Centers Consortium. As part of her faculty role, Ms. Leonardo is a manager of one of the Duquesne University School of Nursing Nurse-Managed Wellness Center sites and is its primary practitioner, working with older adults and precepting undergraduate and graduate students. In addition, she has direct responsibility, along with the director of the nurse-managed wellness center, for all planning, activities, and financial arrangements for the NMWC. She has a number of publications and presentations on this and related topics. In her faculty role, she is the chairperson for BSN Program Committee, which oversees program and curricular issues in the undergraduate program.

Esther Levine-Brill, PhD, ANP-BC

Dr. Esther Levine-Brill is a professor of nursing at Long Island University, Brooklyn Campus in Brooklyn, New York. She teaches in both the undergraduate and graduate programs and is currently chairperson for the undergraduate program. Additionally, she is co-director of the Harriet Rothkopf Heilbrunn B'32 Academic Nursing Center. The center focuses on wellness promotion and prevention for students, faculty, and staff of the Brooklyn campus, as well as for the residents of the surrounding community. She has presented nationally about the nursing center at conferences, as well as locally in her community about various areas related to nursing, curriculum, and the Gulf War call-up, of which she is a veteran.

Rita J. Lourie, RN, MSN, MPH

Ms. Rita Lourie has been the director of academic and community outreach since the inception of Temple Health Connection in 1994, and she has been an assistant professor of nursing at Temple University since 1979. She received her BSN from Alfred University, Alfred, NY; her MSN from University of Texas in El Paso; and her MPH from Temple University. Recently retired, Ms. Lourie is a consultant to the center's director (Dr. Nancy Rothman) and an adjunct faculty member. She is an active member of the public health nurses section and immediate past president of the Philadelphia Hadassah Nurses Council.

Mary Ellen T. Miller, PhD, RN

Dr. Mary Ellen Miller is an assistant professor at De Sales University School of Nursing in Center Valley, Pennsylvania, and teaches in the undergraduate and graduate programs. Dr. Miller serves as the co-chair of the Wellness Center Committee of the National Nursing Center Consortium. She is also co-director of a federal grant at La Salle University Neighborhood Nursing Center, located in Philadelphia, Pennsylvania, where she served as the associate director of public health programs and Independence Foundation chair for three years.

Dr. Miller received her diploma from Chestnut Hill Hospital School of Nursing and a bachelor of science in nursing degree and master's of science in nursing within the public health nursing track from La Salle University. She earned a PhD in health studies from Temple University. Her research interests focus on adolescent and paternal risk communication. She has published about nurse-managed centers and presented regionally and nationally on topics related to her work in this area, as well as the area of student involvement with community service and learning in nurse-managed wellness centers. Dr. Miller is a member of the American Public Health Association, the American Nurses Association, and Sigma Theta Tau International (Kappa Delta Chapter); and she serves on the advisory board of Gwynedd Mercy Academy High School. Dr. Miller has 25 years of experience as a nurse educator and was the recipient of the Von Allman Award for Teaching Excellence at La Salle University in 1999 and the Service to Chapter Award from the Kappa Delta Chapter of Sigma Theta Tau in 2006.

Lisa Ann Plowfield, PhD, RN

Dr. Lisa Ann Plowfield currently serves as dean and professor in the College of Nursing at Florida State University. Formerly, she was the director of the University of Delaware Nursing Center for 10 years and served as one of the founding members of the National Nursing Centers Consortium Advisory Board. During her tenure as director, the UD Nursing Center provided multidisciplinary, comprehensive geriatric assessments for frail older adults throughout Delaware, with an emphasis on older adults in northern Delaware. Numerous programs were funded through state contracts, federal grants, and private funding that offered greatly needed health services and social support to older adults. A major emphasis of all programs was to assist older adults and their family members to access health services to support their care needs. The UD Nursing Center served as a service-learning program for undergraduate and graduate students and as a faculty practice and scholarship initiative. Dr. Plowfield's expertise provided the UD Nursing Center with administrative support, leadership, and an emphasis on family-centered care and family caregiving. Dr. Plowfield continues to consult with UD Nursing Center program staff and to publish outcomes related to the work of the center. Dr. Plowfield received her BSN from Thomas Jefferson University, an MS in nursing from the

University of Maryland, and a PhD in nursing from the University of Virginia. She served on the faculty of the University of Delaware from 1993 to 2007.

Lenore (Leni) Kolljeski Resick, PhD, CRNP, FNP-BC, NP-C

Dr. Leni Resick is an associate professor and director of the Nurse-Managed Wellness Center (DUSON NMWC) and coordinator of the Family Nurse Practitioner Clinical Specialty, Master of Science in Nursing program at Duquesne University School of Nursing in Pittsburgh, Pennsylvania. In 1994, she established the DUSON NMWC at the K. Leroy Irvis Towers site located in the Hill District community of Pittsburgh. She has maintained a practice at the Irvis Towers site as a family nurse practitioner for over 14 years. Dr. Resick is a full-time faculty member and teaches in the undergraduate, master's, and doctoral nursing program at Duquesne University.

Dr. Resick received her diploma from Presbyterian-University Hospital School of Nursing, a bachelor in science in nursing degree and an MSN as a family nurse practitioner from the University of Pittsburgh. She earned a post-master's certificate in transcultural nursing and a PhD in nursing from Duquesne University. Her research interests focus on the meaning of health and wellness for vulnerable, aging, American-born and immigrant/refugee populations. She has published about the Duquesne University Nurse-Managed Centers and presented regionally, nationally, and internationally on topics related to her work with the nurse-managed wellness centers.

Currently Dr. Resick serves on the board of directors of the National Nursing Centers Consortium and the board of directors of the National Organization of Nurse Practitioner Faculties. She is also a member of the American Academy of Nurse Practitioners, the American Nurses Association, and Sigma Theta Tau International (Eta and Epsilon Phi Chapters).

Recently, Dr. Resick was the recipient of the Distinguished Nurse Award given by the Pennsylvania State Nurses Association in recognition of outstanding contributions to the Pennsylvania State Nurses Association members and friends of nursing. She also received the Richard A. Caliguiri Community Action Award given by District 6 of the Pennsylvania State Nurses Association, in recognition of her community practice and international work.

Nancy Rothman, EdD, RN

Dr. Nancy Rothman is the Independence Foundation Professor of Urban Community Nursing in the Department of Nursing, College of Health Professions of Temple University, where she serves as director of community-based practices and oversees an academic wellness center, Temple Health Connection. Her research focuses on community-defined health risks and prevention/intervention strategies for the underserved population. She is the evaluator on most National Nursing Centers Consortium (NNCC) projects and serves as chair of the NNCC Quality Assurance and Research Committee. She serves as a consultant to the Public Health Management Corporation Nursing Network, a network of four primary care centers.

Susan Sims-Giddens, EdD, RN

Dr. Susan Sims-Giddens is an associate professor in the Department of Nursing, Missouri State University. She received her BSN from West Texas A&M, Canyon, Texas; MSN from the University of Texas El Paso; MEd in Bilingual Multicultural Education from Northern Arizona University, Flagstaff, Arizona; and EdD in Educational Leadership from Northern Arizona University. Research interests include academic achievement and educational access for at-risk students, community engagement of nursing students through service learning, a conceptual framework for nursing education, student peer-mentoring, and nurses' and nursing students' attitudes and beliefs about poverty. Dr. Sims-Giddens teaches in an undergraduate generic BSN and BSN completion program, and in the graduate MSN Nurse Educator program.

Donna L. Torrisi, MSN

Ms. Donna Torrisi is the network executive director of the Family Practice & Counseling Network (FPCN), located in Philadelphia, Pennsylvania. She graduated from Villanova University with a BSN in 1972. She received her MSN in 1976 from the University of Pennsylvania as a family nurse-practitioner. In 1991, she cowrote a National Bureau of Primary Health Care/Health Resources Service Administration (HRSA) grant to provide health care to residents of Philadelphia public housing. She became the director of this project and opened a nurse-managed health center in the Abbottsford public housing development in Philadelphia in 1992. Since then, the FPCN has received three expansion grants, in 1994, 2002, and 2003. The three network sites currently serve over 10,000 primarily low-income people with primary care, behavioral health, and oral health care services. The FPCN has received multiple awards, including the HRSA National Models that Work Award and the Smith Kline Beecham Community Impact Award. Ms. Torrisi received the Villanova University Leadership in Nursing award, the University of Pennsylvania Lillian Brunner Sholstis Award for Excellence in Nursing Practice; the Pennsylvania Nurses Association Leadership Award for Innovative Practice; and the National Alliance for Resident Services in Affordable and Assisted Housing, Practitioner of the Year Award.

Ms. Torrisi was a key leader in the movement in the state of Pennsylvania that culminated in legislative change redefining primary care providers to include nurse-practitioners. This gave nurse-practitioners entrée into managed care as participating providers. She has published and lectured on the nurse-managed model, the art of negotiating with managed-care organizations, and integrating behavioral health and primary care. She is a founding member and the first chairperson of the National Nursing Centers Consortium and has been a faculty member for the Institute for Health Improvement Depression Collaborative and the Community Health Center Executive Fellowship Program. Her book, *Community and Nurse-Managed Health Centers: Getting Them Started and Keeping Them Going*, coauthored with Tine Hansen-Turton, was published in May 2005. Donna is a 2005 graduate of the Robert Wood Johnson Executive

Nurse Fellowship program. She currently serves on the Governor's Commission for Chronic Care Management.

M. Elaine Tagliareni, EdD, RN

Dr. M. Elaine Tagliareni is currently a professor of nursing and the Independence Foundation Chair in Community Health Nursing Education in the Nursing Department at Community College of Philadelphia. She has been an associate degree nursing educator for over 25 years. She received her BSN from Georgetown University School of Nursing; a master's degree in mental health and community nursing from the University of California, San Francisco; and her doctorate from Teachers College, Columbia University, with an emphasis on the role of the nurse educator in community colleges.

Since 1995, Dr. Tagliareni has been involved with the design and development of a community-based service-learning project at Community College of Philadelphia. The project is called the 19130 Zip Code Project, funded by the Independence Foundation, Philadelphia, Pennsylvania. Based on outcomes from this project, nursing faculty at the college have developed national conferences to highlight community-based curriculum models and to refocus associate degree nursing education away from a totally acute-care, hospital-based model. Dr. Tagliareni has continued to organize workshops designed to assist faculty to replicate lessons learned from this project, develop data collection methods to describe types of services offered in health-promotion centers, increase retention, and promote critical thinking based on a foundation of co-learner relationships with students. This approach to teaching and learning was one of the primary reasons that the Nursing Department at Community College of Philadelphia was recently honored as a National League for Nursing Center of Excellence.

Currently (2007–2009), Dr. Tagliareni is president of the National League for Nursing (NLN) and is a member of the NLN Board of Governors. Through her wide-ranging participation in NLN committees, she has played a key role in fostering innovation and in promoting the nurse-educator role as an advanced practice role. As president, she hopes to continue to advocate for excellence in nursing education through pedagogical research and to promote dialogue about successful strategies to prepare a diverse nursing workforce.

Roberta Waite, EdD, RN, PMHCNS-BC

Dr. Roberta Waite is an assistant professor at Drexel University in the College of Nursing and Health Professions and a research scientist at the Eleventh Street Family Health Services. Dr. Waite has been a nurse for the past 20 years in varied capacities: clinician, administrator, academician, and researcher. She has a specialized interest in promoting mental health among vulnerable populations, most recently focusing on the process of care of women with depression, adult ADHD among young adults, and developing trauma-informed services within primary health care settings.

References

Chapter 2: What Is a Nurse-Managed Wellness Center?

Eunice King, PhD, RN
Lenore K. Resick, PhD, CRNP, FNP-BC, NP-C

Aydelotte, M. K., Barger, S. E., Branstetter, E., Fehring, R. J., Lindgren, K., Lundeen, S., et al. (1987). *The nursing center: Concept and design*. Kansas City, MO: American Nurses Association.

Clear, J. B., Starbecker, M. M., & Kelly, D. W. (1999). Nursing centers and health promotion: A federal vantage point. *Family and Community Health, 21*(4), 1–14.

U.S. Department of Health and Human Services, Division of Nursing. (2000). *Resource and information guide*. Rockville, MD: Author.

Glass, L. K. (1989). The historical origins of nursing centers. In National League for Nursing (Ed.), *Nursing centers: Meeting the demand for quality healthcare* (pp. 21–34). New York: National League for Nursing.

Hansen-Turton, T., & Kinsey, K. (2001). The quest for self-sustainability: Nurse-managed health centers meeting the policy challenge. *Policy, Politics, & Nursing Practice, 2*(4), 304–309.

Health Resources and Services Administration, Bureau of Health Professions, Division of Nursing. (n.d.). *50 years at the Division of Nursing, United States Public Health Service*. Retrieved September 3, 2003, from http://www.bhpr.hrsa.gov/nursing/50years.htm

King, E. (2005). *Nurse-managed health care funding initiative: History, accomplishments, and current status*. Unpublished report submitted to the Independence Foundation Board of Directors.

King, E. (2008). A 10-year review of four academic nurse-managed centers: Challenges and survival strategies. *Journal of Professional Nursing, 24*(1), 14–20.

Resick, L. K., Taylor, C. A., & Leonardo, M. E. (1999). The nurse-managed wellness clinic model developed by Duquesne University School of Nursing. *Home Health Care Management, 11*(6), 26–35.

Starbecker, M. M. (2000, September). *Historical perspective of Division of Nursing Legislation: 1956–1998*. Paper presented at the Health Resources and Services Administration, Division of Nursing, Nurse-Managed Centers Grantee Meeting, Chevy Chase, MD.

Tagliareni, E., & King, E. (2006). Documenting health promotion services in community-based nursing centers. *Holistic Nursing Practice, 20*(1), 20–26.

Torrisi, D. L., & Hansen-Turton, T. (2005). *Community and nurse-managed health centers: Getting them started and keeping them going* (pp. 1–10). New York: Springer Publishing Company.

United States Department of Health and Human Services. (2005, January). *Healthy people 2010: The cornerstone for prevention*. Rockville, MD: Author. Retrieved July 13, 2008, from http://www.healthypeople.gov/Publications

United States Department of Health and Human Services. (1991) *Healthy people 2000: National health promotion and disease prevention objectives* (Publication No. PHS 91–50213). Washington, DC: Public Health Service.

Chapter 3: Application of the Boyer Model of Scholarship in Nurse-Managed Wellness Centers

Lenore K. Resick, PhD, CRNP, FNP-BC, NP-C
Maureen E. Leonardo, MN, CRNP, CNE, FNP-BC

American Association of Critical Care Nurses. (n.d.). *The synergy model for patient care.* Retrieved May 2, 2008, from http://web.aacn.org/DesktopModules/Certifications/pages/Certifications/general/synmodel.aspx

Boyer, E. L. (1990). *Scholarship reconsidered: Priorities of the professoriate.* Princeton, NJ: The Carnegie Foundation for the Advancement of Teaching.

Fiandt, K., Laux, C. A., Sarver, N. L., & Sayer, R. J. (2002). Finding the nurse in nurse practitioner practice: A pilot study of rural family nurse practitioner practice. *Clinical Excellence for Nurse Practitioner, 5*(6), 13–30.

Glassick, C. E., Huber, M. T., & Maeroff, G. I. (1997). *Scholarship assessed: Evaluation of the professoriate.* San Francisco: Jossey-Bass.

Nibert, M. (n.d.). *Boyer's Model of Scholarship.* Retrieved March 13, 2008, from http://www.pcrest.com/PC/FGB/test/2_5_1.htm

Chapter 4: Organizational Development

Philip Greiner

Barger, S. (1995). Establishing a nursing center: Learning from the literature and the experiences of others. *Journal of Professional Nursing, 11*(4), 203–212.

CDC. (2008). *Clinical Laboratory Improvement Amendments (CLIA).* Retrieved July 7, 2008, from http://wwwn.cdc.gov/clia/default.aspx

U. S. Small Business Administration. (2008). *Small Business Planner.* Retrieved July 19, 2008, from http://www.sba.gov/smallbusinessplanner/plan/writeabusinessplan/index.html

Value-added. (2008). In *Merriam-Webster Online Dictionary.* Retrieved July 8, 2008, from http://www.merriam-webster.com/dictionary/value-added

Chapter 5: Planning a Wellness Center

Maureen Leonardo, MN, CRNP, CNE, FNP-BC
Lenore K. Resick, PhD, CRNP, FNP-BC, NP-C
Donna Torrisi, MSN
Tine Hansen-Turton, MGA
Ann Deinhardt, MSW

Buppert, C. (2004). *Nurse practitioner's business practice and legal guide* (2nd ed.). Sudbury, MA: Jones and Bartlett.

Clemen-Stone, S., McGuire, S. L., & Eigsti, D. G. (2002). *Comprehensive community health nursing: Family, aggregate, & community practice* (6th ed.). Philadelphia: Mosby.

Esposito, C. L. (2000). What's the point of malpractice insurance? *Nursing Spectrum, 12*(13), 6–7.

Hunt, R. (2009). *Introduction to community-based nursing.* Philadelphia: Wolters Kluwer/Lippincott Williams & Wilkins.

McNamara, C. (n.d.). *Basics of conducting focus groups.* Retrieved July 12, 2008, from http://www.managementhelp.org/evaluatn/focusgrp.htm

U.S. Small Business Administration. (n.d.). *Write a business plan*. Retrieved June 5, 2008, from http://www.sba.gov/smallbusinessplanner/plan/writeabusinessplan/index.html

Chapter 6: Community Presence and Marketing

Esther Levine-Brill, PhD, APRN-BC
Rita Lourie, RN, MSN, MPH
Mary Ellen Miller, MSN, RN

Rothman, N. L., Lourie, R. J., Dyer, A., & Gass, D. L. (2000). A successful community-based partnership: Formation and achievements. *Metropolitan University: An International Forum, 11,* 59–62.

Chapter 7: Funding and Sustainability of Wellness Centers

Philip A. Greiner, DNSc, RN

Barger, S. (1995). Establishing a nursing center: Learning from the literature and the experiences of others. *Journal of Professional Nursing, 11*(4), 203–212.

Chapter 10: Wellness Center Services for Aging Populations

Diane Haleem, PhD, RN

American Heart Association, Inc. (2002). *The national high blood pressure education program, thirty years and counting, an editorial*. Retrieved August 2008 from hyper.ahajournals. org/cgi/content/full/39/5/941

Centers for Disease Control. (2008). *Seasonal flu shot*. Retrieved July 6, 2008, from http://www. cdc. gov/flu/about/qa/flushot.htm

Federal Interagency Forum on Aging-Related Statistics. (2008). *Older Americans 2008: Key indicators of well-being*. Retrieved August 2008 from http://agingstats.gov/agingstatsdotnet/ MainSite/Data/2008Documents/Health_Risks.aspx

National Agricultural Library, Food and Nutrition Information Center. (2007). *General nutrition resource list for older adults*. Retrieved August 2008 from www.nal.usda.gov/fnic/pubs/ olderadults.pdf

U.S. Department of Commerce, Economics and Statistics Administration, Bureau of the Census. (1993). *We the American elderly*. Retrieved August 2008 from www.census. gov/apsd/wepeople/we-9.pdf

U.S. Department of Health and Human Services. National Institutes of Health, National Heart, Lung, and Blood Institute, National High Blood Pressure Program. (2004). *Prevent and control high blood pressure: Mission possible*. Retrieved August 2008 from http://hp2010. nhlbihin.net/mission/partner/midlife.pdf

U.S. Department of Health and Human Services, National Institute of Diabetes and Digestive and Kidney Diseases. (2004) *Weight-control information network*. Retrieved August 2008 from http://win.niddk.nih.gov/statistics/index.htm

U.S. Department of Health and Human Services, Food and Drug Administration. (2006). *Eating well as we age*. Retrieved August 2008 from http://www.fda.gov/opacom/lowlit/eatage.html

U.S. Department of Health and Human Services, Public Health Service, National Institutes of Health, National Institute on Aging, Reprinted April 2008. *Exercise: A guide from the National Institute on Aging*. Retrieved August 2008 from http://www.niapublications.org/ exercisebook/ExerciseGuideComplete.pdf

Chapter 11: Wellness Center Services for Latino Populations

Julie Cousler Emig

Alegría, M., Mulvaney-Day, N., Torres, M., Polo, A., Cao, Z., & Canino, G. (2007). Prevalence of psychiatric disorders across Latino subgroups in the United States. *American Journal of Public Health, 97,* 68–75.

Child Trends. (2008). *Facts at a glance: a fact sheet reporting national, state-level, and city-level trends in teen childbearing* (Publication #2008-29). Retrieved August 2008 from http://www.childtrends.org/files/Child_Trends-2008_07_30_FactsAtAGlance.pdf

Harralson, T. L., Cousler Emig, J., Polansky, M., Walker, R., Otero-Cruz, J., & Garcia-Leeds, C. (2007). Un corazon saludable: Factors influencing outcomes of an exercise program designed to impact cardiac and metabolic risks among urban Latinas. *Journal for Community Health, 32,* 401–412.

Hecht, M., & Marsiglia, F. (1989). *keepin' It REAL (Refuse, Explain, Avoid, Leave) Curriculum.* The Pennsylvania State University, PA.

Jemmott, L., Jemmott, J., III, & McCaffree, K. (1989). *Be Proud! Be Responsible! Curriculum.* New York: Select Media, Inc.

Pennsylvania Coalition Against Domestic Violence. (2006). *JARS (Justice, Accountability, Responsibility, Safety) curriculum.* PCADV. Harrisburg, PA.

Pew Hispanic Center: Pew Research Center. (2006). *Statistical portrait of Hispanics in the United States, 2006.* Retrieved June 25, 2008, from www.pewhispanic.org/factsheets/factsheet.php?FactsheetID=35

U.S. Census Bureau, Population Division. (2006). *Hispanics in the United States.* Retrieved July 1, 2008, from www.census.gov/population/www/socdemo/hispanic/hispanic.html

U.S. Department of Health and Human Services, Centers for Disease Control and Prevention, Office of Enterprise Communication. (2008). *Nation's high school students showing overall improvements in health-related behaviors; However, Hispanic students not showing progress in some key areas.* Press release dated July 2008.

U.S. Department of Health and Human Services, Centers for Disease Control and Prevention, Divisions of HIV/AIDS Prevention, National Center for HIV/AIDS, Viral Hepatitis, STD, and TB Prevention. (2008). *HIV/AIDS among Hispanics/Latinos.* Retrieved August 2008 from www.cdc.gov/hiv/hispanics

Chapter 12: Mental Health Services in Wellness Centers

Donna L. Torrisi, MSN, CRNP
Penny Killian, MSN, RN, PNP
Roberta Waite, EdD, RN, PMHCNS-BC

Cole, S., & Cole, M. R. (2002, January). *Depression in chronic medical illness: Assessment, management, tools, and care coordination.* Paper presented at The Bureau of Primary Care: Health Disparities Collaboratives, Chicago, IL.

De Groot, M., Anderson, R., Freeland, K., Clouse, R., & Lustman, P. (2001). Association of depression and diabetes complications: A meta-analysis. *Psychosomatic Medicine, 63,* 619–630.

Depression Guideline Panel. (1993). Depression in primary care: Detection, diagnosis, and treatment. *Quick Reference Guide for Clinicians, Number 5* (AHCPR Publication No. 93-0552, April). Rockville, MD: U.S. Department of Health and Human Services, Public Health Service, Agency for Health Care Policy and Research.

Hauenstein, E. (1996). Testing innovative nursing care: Home interventions with depressed rural women. *Issues in Mental Health Nursing, 17,* 33–50.

Institute for Health Improvement. (2002). Depression: Changing Practice, Changing Lives. *Depression, the Challenge, 4.*

Lyons-Ruth, K., Connell, D., Grunebaum, H., & Botein, S. (1990). Infants at social risk: Maternal depression and family support services as mediators of infant development and security and attachment. *Child Development, 61,* 85–98.

Myers, J. E., Sweeny, T. J., & Witmer, J. M. (2000). The wheel of wellness counseling for wellness: A holistic model for treatment planning. *Journal of Counseling and Development, 78*, 251–266.

National Nursing Centers Consortium. (2000). *Data mart project.* Unpublished manuscript.

U.S. Department of Health and Human Services. (1999). *Mental Health: A Report of the Surgeon General.* Rockville, MD: U.S. Department of Health and Human Services, Substance Abuse and Mental Health Services Administration, Center for Mental Health Services, National Institutes of Health, National Institute of Mental Health.

Chapter 13: Community Service and Learning and Student Engagement

Evelyn Hayes, PhD, APRN, BC

Diane Haleem, PhD, RN

Joan Miller, PhD, CRNP, FNP-C

Mary Ellen Miller, PhD, RN

Lisa Plowfield, PhD, RN

American Association of Colleges of Nursing. (2008). *Nursing shortage fact sheet.* Retrieved July 13, 2008, from http://www.aacn.nche.edu/ Media/FactSheets/NursingShortage.htm

Astin, L., & Sax, A. (1998). How undergraduates are affected by service participation. *Journal of College Student Development, 39*, 251–263.

Bentley, R., & Ellison, J. (2005). Impact of a service-learning project on nursing students. *Nursing Education Perspectives, 26*, 287–290.

Butin, D. W. (2003). Of what use is it? Multiple conceptualizations of service learning within education. *Teachers College Review, 105*, 1674–1692.

Champagne, N. (2006). Service learning: Its origin, evolution, and connection to health education. *American Journal of Health Education, 37*, 97–101.

Clear, J. B., Starbecker, M. M., & Kelly, D. W. (1999). Nursing centers and health promotion: A federal vantage point. *Family and Community Health, 21*(4), 1–14.

Cushman, E. (2002). Sustainable service learning programs. *College Composition and Communication, 54*, 40–65.

Eyler, J., & D. E. Giles, J. (1999). *Where's the learning in service-learning?* San Francisco: Jossey-Bass.

Eyler, J., D. E. Giles, J., Stenson, C., & Gray, C. (2001). *At a glance: What we know about the effects of service-learning on college students, faculty, institutions, and communities, 1993–2000.* Vanderbilt University: Corporation for National Service Learn and Serve America National Service Learning Clearinghouse. Nashville, TN.

Foss, G. F., Bonaiuto, M. M., Johnson, Z. S., & Moreland, D. M. (2003). Using Polvika's model to create a service-learning partnership. *Journal of School Health, 73*, 305–310.

Harrington, P. (1999). Integrating service-learning into the curriculum. In P. A. Bailey, D. R. Carpenter, & P. A. Harrington (Eds.), *Integrating community service into nursing education: A guide to service-learning.* New York: Springer.

Long, A. B., Larsen, P., Hussey, L., & Travis, S. S. (2001). Organizing, managing, and evaluating service-learning projects. *Educational Gerontology, 27*, 3–21.

Mercer, D. K., & Brungardt, C. (2007, June 22). Case study: Institutionalizing service-learning at Fort Hays University. *National Civic Review*, p. 54.

Miller, M. E., & Giugliano, L. (2006, September 22). The real world: Service, learning and missions. *Academic Exchange Quarterly, 10*(3), 30–34.

National Service Learning Clearinghouse. (2008). *What is service learning.* Retrieved July 14, 2008, from http://www.servicelearning.org/what_is_service-learning/service-learning_is/index

Newman, M. A. (2003). A world of no boundaries. *Advances in Nursing Science, 26*(4), 240–245.

Patton, R. M. (2007). Move over – This generation is ready. *The American Nurse, 40*, 4.

Sedlak, C. A., Doheny, M. O., Panthofer, N., & Anaya, E. (2003). Critical thinking in students' service-learning experiences. *College Teaching, 51*, 99–103.

Shaw, H. K., & Degazon, C. (2008). Integrating the core professional vales of nursing: A profession, not just a career. *Journal of Cultural Diversity, 15*, 44–50.

Sigmon, R. (1979). Service learning: Three principles. *Synergist, 8*, 9–11.

Sigmon, R. (1994). Serving to learn, learning to serve. In *Linking service with learning in liberal arts education*. Washington, DC: Council of Independent Colleges.

Steinke, P., & Fitch, P. (2007). Assessing service learning. *Research and Practice in Assessment, 1*, 1–8.

Chapter 14: Extending the Mission of Wellness Centers to Build Future Nursing Capacity

Evelyn Hayes, PhD, APRN, BC

Lisa Plowfield, PhD, RN

Diane Haleem, PhD, RN

Joan Miller, PhD, CRNP, FNP-C

Mary Ellen Miller, PhD, RN

American Association of Colleges of Nursing. (2008). *The essentials of baccalaureate education: For professional practice*. Washington, DC: Author.

Dunham, K. S. & Smith, S. J. (2005). *How to survive and maybe even love your life as a nurse*. Philadelphia: F.A. Davis.

MinorityNurse.com. (2000). *Minority nursing statistics*. Retrieved July 13, 2008, from http://www.minoritynurse.com/statistics.html

Sherrod, B. (2005, September). Men at work. *Nursing Management, 36*(9), 74–75.

United States Department of Labor Statistics. (2007, November). *Monthly Labor Review*. Washington, DC: U.S. Dept. of Labor.

Chapter 15: Measuring Quality in Wellness Centers

Susan M. Hinck, PhD, RN

Baicker, K., & Chandra, A. (2004). Medicare spending, the physician workforce, and beneficiaries' quality of care. *Health Affairs Web Exclusives Supplement, W4*, 184–197.

Berwick, D. M., Nolan, T. W., & Whittington, J. (2008). The triple aim: Care, health, and cost. *Health Affairs, 27*, 759–769.

Coddington, J. A., & Sands, L. P. (2008). Cost of health care and quality outcomes of patients at nurse-managed clinics. *Nursing Economics, 26*, 75–83.

Corrigan, J. (2007). *Tracking NQF-endorsed consensus standards for nursing-sensitive care: A 15-month study*. Washington, DC: National Quality Forum.

Institute of Medicine. (2001). *Crossing the quality chasm: A new health system for the 21st century*. Washington, DC: National Academies Press.

Institute of Medicine. (2006a). *Medicare's quality improvement organization program: Maximizing potential*. Washington, DC: National Academies Press.

Institute of Medicine. (2006b). *Performance measurement: Accelerating improvement*. Washington, DC: National Academies Press.

Institute of Medicine. (2007). *Rewarding provider performance: Aligning incentives in Medicare*. Washington, DC: National Academies Press.

McGlynn, E. A., Asch, S. M., Adams, J., Keesey, J., Hicks, J., DeCristofaro, A., et al. (2003). The quality of health care delivered to adults in the United States. *New England Journal of Medicine, 348*, 2635–2645.

MedPac. (2006). *Report to Congress: Increasing the value of Medicare*. Retrieved April 5, 2008, from http//:www.medPAC.gov/documents/Jun06_EntireReport.pdf

Montalvo, I. (2007, September 30). The National Database of Nursing Quality Indicators (NDNQI). *The Online Journal of Issues in Nursing: A Scholarly Journal of the ANA, 12*(3). Retrieved February 13, 2008, from http://nursingworld.org/MainMenuCategories/ANA Marketplace/ANA Periodicals/OJIN/TableofContents/Volume122007/No3Sept07/Nurs ingQualityIndicators.aspx

Murphy, B. (Ed.). (1995). *Nursing centers: The time is now*. New York: National League for Nursing Press.

O'Kane, M., Corrigan, J., Foote, S. M., Tunis, S. R., Isham, G. J., Nichols, L. M., et al. (2008). Crossroads in Quality. *Health Affairs, 27*, 749–758.

Rantz, M., Bostick, J., & Riggs, C. J. (2002). *Nursing quality measurement: A review of nursing studies 1995–2000*. Washington, DC: American Nurses Publishing.

Wennberg, J. E., Fisher, E. S., & Skinner, J. S. (2002). Geography and the debate over Medicare reform. *Health Affairs Web Exclusives Supplement, W2*, 96–114.

Chapter 16: Documenting Outcomes

Lenore K. Resick, PhD, CRNP, FNP-BC, NP-C
Evelyn Hayes, PhD, APRN, BC
Maureen E. Leonardo, MN, CRNP, CNE, FNP-BC
Lisa Plowfield, PhD, RN

American Medical Association. (2008). *Current procedural terminology*. Retrieved July 19, 2008, from http://www.ama-assn.org/ama/pub/category/3113.html

Christensen, J. R., Koudos, C. E., & Clark, J. (2005). Omaha System experiences in practice: Documenting Sure Start services in Wales. In K. S. Martin, *The Omaha system: Key to practice, documentation, and information management* (pp. 79–80). St. Louis, MO: Elsevier.

Dochterman, J. M., & Bulechek, G.M. (Eds.). (2004). *Nursing interventions classification (NIC)* (4th ed.). St. Louis, MO: Mosby.

Lampe, S. (1997). *Focus Charting documentation for patient-centered care* (7th ed.). Minneapolis: Creative HealthCare Management.

Leonardo, M. E., Resick, L. K., Bingman, C., & Strotmeyer, S. (2004). The alternatives for wellness centers: Drown in data or develop a reasonable electronic documentation system. *Home Heath Care Management & Practice, 16*(3), 177–184.

Martin, K. S., & Scheet, N. J. (1992). *The Omaha system: Applications for community health nursing*. Philadelphia: Saunders.

Moorhead, S., Johnson, M., & Maas, M. (Eds.). (2004). *Nursing outcome classification (NOC)* (3rd ed.). St. Louis: Mosby.

Norusis, M. (2002). *SPSS 11.0 guide to data analysis*. Upper Saddle River, NJ: Prentice Hall.

Resick, L. K., Taylor, C., & Leonardo, M. E. (1999). The nurse-managed wellness clinic model developed by Duquesne University School of Nursing. *Home Health Care Management & Practice, 11*(6), 26–35.

Taylor, C., Resick, L. K., D'Antonio, J. A., & Carroll, T. L. (1997). The advanced practice nurse role in implementing and evaluating two nurse-managed wellness clinics: Lessons learned about structure, process, and outcomes. *Advanced Practice Quarterly, 3*(2), 36–45.

Wade, D. T. (2004). Assessment, measurement, and data collection tools. *Clinical Rehabilitation, 18*(3), 233–237.

Weiss, D. M., Schank, M. J., Coenen, A., & Matheus, R. (2002). Parish nurse practice with client aggregates. *Journal of Community Health Nursing, 19*(2), 105–113.

Chapter 17: Data Collection

Eunice S. King, PhD, RN
M. Elaine Tagliareni, EdD, RN

Anderko, L. & Kinion, E. (2001). Speaking with a unified voice: Recommendations for the collection of aggregated outcome data in nursing centers. *Policy, Politics, & Nursing Practice, 2*, 295–303.

Deshefy-Longhi, T., Swartz, M. K., & Grey, M. (2008). Characterizing nurse practitioner practice by sampling patient encounters: An APRNet study. *Journal of the American Academy of Nurse Practitioners, 20*, 281–287.

Lundeen, S. P. (1999). An alternative paradigm for promoting health in communities: The Lundeen Community Nursing Center model. *Family and Community Health, 21*, 15–28.

Martin, K., Leak, G., & Aden, C. (1997). The Omaha system: A research-based model for decision-making. In B.W. Spradley & J.A. Allender (Eds.), *Teachings in community health nursing* (5th ed., pp. 316–324). Philadelphia: Lippincott-Raven.

National Nursing Center Consortium Programs. (2005). *Lead safe babies and asthma safe kids.* Retrieved August 1, 2005, from www.nncc.us/programs

Rothman, N., Lourie, R., & Gaughan, J. (2002). Lead awareness: North Philly style. *American Journal of Public Health, 92*, 739–941.

Tagliareni, M., & King, E. (2006, January/February). Documenting health promotion services in community-based nursing centers. *Holistic Nursing Practice, 20*(1), 20–26.

U.S. Department of Health and Human Services (USDHHS). (2000). *Healthy people 2010: Understanding and improving health* (2nd ed.). Washington, DC: U.S. Government Printing Office.

Appendix A

University of Delaware Nursing Center–Newark, Delaware
Roosevelt, Franklin Delano. Inaugural Address. January 20, 1937.

Appendix B

Integrated Health Care–Chicago, Illinois
McDevitt, J., Braun, S., Noyes, M., Snyder, M., & Marion, L. (2005, December). Integrated primary and mental health care: Evaluating a nurse-managed center for patients with serious and persistent mental illness. *Nursing Clinics of North America, 40*(4), 779–790, xii.

Appendix C

La Salle Neighborhood Nursing Center–Philadelphia, Pennsylvania
American Academy of Pediatrics, American Public Health Association, National Resource Center for Health and Safety in Child Care, National Health and Safety Performance Standards, 2002, p. 32.

Index

CPSIA information can be obtained at www.ICGtesting.com
Printed in the USA
BVOW021127230413

318898BV00003B/47/P